RA395.C^ ---- ----

0134

Impleme
  care
    c2

2006 02 27

Implementing
Primary
Care
Reform

Barriers and Facilitators

Implementing
Primary
Care
Reform

Barriers and Facilitators

Edited by
Ruth Wilson, S.E.D. Shortt and John Dorland

Published for the School of Policy Studies
by McGill-Queen's University Press
Montreal & Kingston • London • Ithaca

National Library of Canada Cataloguing in Publication

Implementing primary care reform : barriers and facilitators / edited by Ruth Wilson, S.E.D. Shortt and John Dorland.

Papers originally presented at a conference held Nov. 2-4, 2003 in Kingston, Ont. Conference initiated by the Ontario Family Health Network, and organized in partnership with the School of Policy Studies with assistance from the Queen's Centre for Health Services and Policy Research, and the Queen's Centre for Studies in Primary Care.
Includes bibliographical references.
ISBN 1-55339-041-5 (bound).—ISBN 1-55339-040-7 (pbk.)

1. Health care reform—Canada—Congresses. 2. Health care reform—Congresses. I. Wilson, Ruth, 1952- II. Shortt, S. E. D. (Samuel Edward Dole), 1947- III. Dorland, John, 1946- IV. Queen's University (Kingston, Ont.). School of Policy Studies

RA393.I46 2004   362.1'0971   C2004-902421-3

Contents

Preface

O n November 2–4, 2003, approximately 100 people from across Canada and around the world met in Kingston, Ontario, to discuss the implementation of primary care reform.

This event was initiated by the Ontario Family Health Network, the agency established by the Government of Ontario to implement primary care reform in the province. It was organized in partnership with the Queen's University School of Policy Studies, with assistance from the Queen's Centre for Health Services and Policy Research, and the Queen's Centre for Studies in Primary Care.

Supporting funding was provided by the Primary Health Care Transition Fund (Health Canada), the Canadian Health Services Research Foundation, and the Ontario Family Health Network.

Impetus for this conference, and this book, which consists of papers written by many of the presenters at the event, stemmed from the following observations:

- Primary care reform is at the heart of Canadian and international health care debates. Two recent major reviews of the Canadian health care system (the Kirby and Romanow reports) devoted large sections to primary care reform, and the recent federal-provincial agreement on health care dedicated significant funding to this purpose.
- Despite the broad consensus on the importance of primary care reform in theory, achieving such reform is proving difficult in practice. In Canada, all provinces and territories have been designing and implementing reforms in primary care. Their approaches to program design, implementation, and pace differ, but nowhere is the process proving to be speedy.
- Canadian federal/provincial/territorial policy-makers and decision makers have a great deal of knowledge to share with each other regarding implementation issues in primary care reform.

This book is a contribution toward the practical work of implementing primary care renewal. Michael Decter leads off with an introduction to the Canadian health policy landscape. The first section, with contributions from S.E.D.Shortt and Raisa Deber, looks at the clinical and economic rationale for reform — why undertake this in the first place? We then examine experience in other countries, both from a policy and practical perspective. Nick Mays and Jackie Cumming describe the New Zealand experience, and Bonnie Sibbald, Rod Sheaff and Martin Roland that of the United Kingdom. Political preconditions for change are described by two political scientists, Carolyn Tuohy and Antonia Maioni. The implications of reform in the Canadian context are discussed by Brian Hutchinson, Marie-Dominique Beaulieu, and Catherine Fooks. Finally, Barbara Starfield provides us with compelling arguments for why overall health outcomes are better with a strong primary care system.

The second part of the book describes recent progress toward primary care reforms from each province in Canada, provided by provincial ministries of health.

We hope you enjoy the rich mix of policy and practicality the authors have brought to this work.

Introduction

Reflections on Primary Care in Canada

Michael Decter

The decade of the 1990s in Canada, as in many other industrialized countries, witnessed the emergence of a central, overwhelming focus in health care reform — the consolidation and the restructuring of the inpatient acute care hospital. In less than a decade we saw radical restructuring of hitherto stand-alone general hospitals into much larger multi-site hospitals and in many cases into full health systems. Most other countries also undertook significant changes to the organization of primary care. Canada, nearly alone among the industrialized, wealthy countries, and no less convinced of the need for change, did not move very far forward in reform of primary care during the 1990s.

I have three fundamental beliefs about primary care:

First, I strongly believe that without a more robust and comprehensive package of primary health care services we will lose the ground gained in the 1990s in health reform. We will simply fail to meet the needs of our citizens.

Second, I believe that the increasing needs of the population for prevention of disease and assistance with the management of chronic disease require more powerful primary care.

Third, I completely believe the real issue in Canada is implementation. There is an abundance of policy work, there is a plethora of Canadian studies dating back over 50 years that are remarkable in their sameness. What we need now are practical actions.

In short, the implementation of primary care reforms must be the central issue to be solved in Canadian health care in this decade. New models or new studies are not the solution, nor will rehashing old debates solve the problem; what is needed to meet the challenge is a lot of energy devoted to issues of implementation.

We need to recognize at the outset that we are dealing with a diverse set of existing arrangements in primary care. Variances are great across provinces, even within provinces. For example, Sault Ste. Marie has a long history of the group health centre and remains an inspirational model of how care can be delivered. But can their history be replicated elsewhere or is it unique to them? Fortunately, we are also not trying to move to a single destination. Primary care services will tend to vary based on factors such as population density, proximity to major centres, and a myriad of other factors. Population density is a confounding factor, not fully appreciated in the effort to move innovative models from one country to another.

We have much to learn from experiences across the great natural experiment that is Canada. Sadly, we have not learned as much as we might from over 30 years of the CLSC experience in the Province of Quebec. There is also much to be learned from recent experience in Ontario with the Ontario Family Health Network. This innovation has improved the access of many, many Ontarians to the primary care services they need.

I have the privilege of serving as chair of the board of the Canadian Institute for Health Information, better known simply as CIHI. In our annual Health Care in Canada Report for 2003 (1) we gave priority to an examination of primary care. We included a full chapter on primary care pulling together data and experience from across Canada. We also devoted a chapter to family doctors. I wish now to review some of our more interesting findings.

PROVIDING PRIMARY CARE

Multiple Providers

The report notes that in descending order of numbers the following 18 professions contributed to primary care in Canada in 2001: registered nurses, social workers, general and family practitioners, dental assistants, pharmacists, dentists, ambulance attendants, psychologists, physiotherapists, dental hygienists, occupational therapists, dieticians/nutritionists, audiologists, dental technicians, opticians, chiropractors, midwives and optometrists. This is a list that underscores the complexity of primary care.

Nurse Practitioners

According to the 2001 National Family Physician Workforce Survey, approximately 7 percent of family doctors who report that their main practice setting is a private

FIGURE 1

CANADA'S PRIMARY HEALTH CARE PROVIDERS

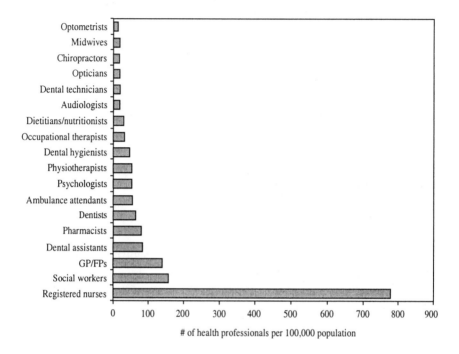

# of health professionals per 100,000 population

FIGURE 2

NURSE PRACTITIONERS WHO WORK WITH FAMILY PHYSICIANS

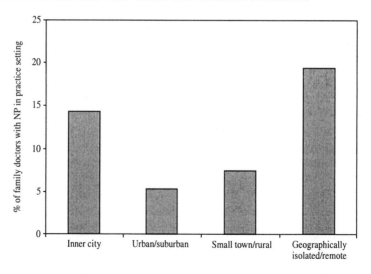

office, community clinic, academic family medicine teaching unit, or free-standing walk-in clinic, said there was a nurse practitioner in that setting. Physicians who practice primarily in inner cities (15 percent) and in remote areas (20 percent) were most likely to report that they worked with nurse practitioners.

Gaps in Care

A point on equity questions. Both medicine and dentistry are rightly part of primary care. Access to doctors has been an insured service since the 1960s. Dental care is still a mix of employer and individual insurance or direct pay. The consequence is that poor Canadians have far worse access to dentists than they do to doctors. Although access has improved for all income groups, the pre-medicare gradient in access to doctors has been eliminated and the gradient for access to dentists — wealthier Canadians have dramatically better access — has been maintained.

Using survey data from 1950/51 and 2000/01, Canadian households were divided into four equally sized income groups. At each income level, in the year 2000/01, Canadians aged 12 and over were more likely to have reported visiting a doctor or dentist in the past year than households were to have reported paying for such services a half century earlier.

Informal Care

Another key point highlighted in the CIHI report is the important role of lending a helping hand or informal care. The formal paid health system perches atop a much larger family and friends network. Over the years we have moved to insure more services in reaction to needs, changing family structure, and popular demand. Yet in 2000, 77 percent of Canadians aged 15 and over reported helping one another on a one-to-one basis. The types of activities that they helped with varied. For example, more men than women reported helping with yard and maintenance work, teaching, and coaching. On the other hand, more women than men reported having helped with housework, babysitting, visiting, and providing direct care to the sick or elderly.

HAVE WE MADE PROGRESS?

In some cases dramatic progress has not received the attention it deserves. For example, I would argue that the broad availability of telehealth or more narrowly

FIGURE 3

USE OF PHYSICIAN AND DENTAL SERVICES

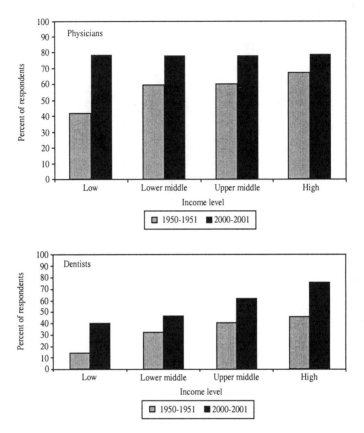

Note: The 1950/51 survey asked respondents about three classes of physician services: "office calls," "home calls," and "clinic visits" during the survey year. Dentist services were classified as "care received by patients from qualified dentists" during visits to "dentists' offices or clinics," including hospital out-patient clinics. The 2000/01 survey asked somewhat different questions of individuals: "Not counting when you were an overnight patient, in the past 12 months, how many times have you seen or talked on the phone, about your physical, emotional or mental health with a family doctor or general practitioner?" The same questions was also asked for dentists or orthodontists.

nurse call-lines represent the addition of an important element to the primary care system. We now need to link telehealth firmly back to provider organizations, as in the case of Capital Health in Edmonton. Another example, as yet to reach Canada, is the addition of electronic prescribing as a universal reality to reduce the significant risks to the health of patients caused by prescribing or

FIGURE 4
LENDING A HELPING HAND

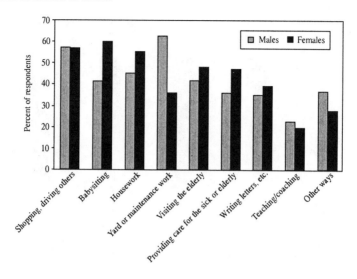

dispensing errors. The United Kingdom and New Zealand have moved rapidly to achieve very high levels of electronic prescribing by family doctors with tangible benefits. Finally, the many multidisciplinary Family Health Network practices are eloquent testimony to successful change.

But such progress notwithstanding, we still are in need of substantial change. I suggest the following barriers to change require urgent attention:

Barrier 1. Inertia
We are all in the habit of doing tomorrow what we did yesterday. This is particularly true in health care. It is difficult but necessary to break the old patterns.

Barrier 2. Absence of a Management Structure
The most significant barrier to movement to reformed primary care is, in my view, the absence of a management structure in much of Family Medicine. Solo practitioners are often too busy doing their work to attend meetings with others to discuss change. It explains in large measure why the reformation of hospitals proved, while challenging, much easier to accomplish. This might be addressed by movement to group practice among family doctors, which would ensure a management structure of some type.

Barrier 3. Centralized Bargaining that Creates, in Some Cases, Barriers to Local Action
There is a need to build-in, at the central table, room for local action and diversity, through flexibility and negotiation.

CONCLUSIONS

I remain an optimist about health care reform in general and about primary care reform in particular. We can do this important thing if we are determined and patient. I know that the essays in this book will advance all of our thinking about how to achieve needed change. The sharing of lessons across borders, including the borders of our own Canadian provinces, is valuable as long as we are careful to fully understand differences in national values and situations. I absolutely believe we will succeed over the next decade in meeting the needs of all Canadians for access to high quality, comprehensive primary care.

REFERENCE

1   Canadian Institute for Health Information. Health Care in Canada. Ottawa; the Institute, 2003 http://www.cihi.ca All figures following are available at http://secure.cihi.ca/cihiweb/dispPage.jsp?cw_page=AR43_2003data_e

Section 1

Setting the Context for Implementing Primary Care Reform

Primary Care Reform
Is There a Clinical Rationale?

S.E.D. Shortt

INTRODUCTION

In White's classic paper of 1961 (1) on the ecology of medical care, and in the recent update of this work by Green et al. (2), the dominant role of primary care in the health systems is clear: the vast majority of formal care consumption occurs at the primary care level. This utilization, in turn, has an important impact on population health status. Barbara Starfield and her colleagues have produced compelling evidence to show the strong correlation in OECD countries between health outcomes and the strength of a country's primary health care system (3). Considerations such as these may have motivated a recent succession of national (4,5) and provincial commissions (6–10) in Canada to argue that health reform must begin with primary care. It is critical, however, that this ubiquitous enthusiasm for primary care reform pay close attention to the evidence upon which proposed innovations are based. The following paper poses the question: Is there a *clinical* rationale for primary care reform in Canada, that is, will proposed changes be likely to enhance the *quality of care*? It will answer the inquiry by first identifying the key elements of primary care reform and then reviewing the existing clinical and health services literature that relates to each of these components.

DEFINING PRIMARY CARE REFORM

While there is no absolute consensus as to what, exactly, constitutes primary care reform in Canada, there are a number of commonly identified components. Table 1 illustrates visions of the concept from four credible sources. For the purposes of the current paper, the key elements of primary care reform and

TABLE 1

COMPONENTS OF PRIMARY CARE REFORM

Primary Health Care Transition Fund (11)	"Romanow" (4)	"Kirby" (5)	Ontario Ministry of Health and Long-Term Care (12)
Service to a defined population	Continuity and coordination of care	Patient rostering	Patient rostering
Increased health promotion and disease prevention	Early detection and action	Health promotion and disease prevention	Illness prevention
Expanded 24/7 access to care		24/7 access to care	24/7 access to care
Multidisciplinary teams		Team of various types of providers	Multidisciplinary teams
Coordinate and integrate with rest of the health care system			
	Enhanced information on need, outcomes	Electronic patient record	Enhanced information technology
	New and stronger incentives	Alternatives to fee-for-service	
			Comprehensive care

their accompanying clinical justifications will be taken to be those presented in Table 2. A review of the existing literature will permit identification of evidence which supports validity of these clinical rationales.

ROSTERED PATIENTS

By having patients formally enlist on the roster of a designated practice it is anticipated that a close bond will form between patients and their care providers. This relationship, in turn, will foster continuity, a core value of contemporary primary care (13). Though elusive to define with precision, continuity is said to be composed of several key elements: an awareness on the provider's part of

TABLE 2

FIVE KEY ELEMENTS AND CLINICAL RATIONALES OF PRIMARY CARE REFORM

Key Element	*Clinical Rationale*
Rostered patients	Closer doctor-patient relationship leading to enhanced continuity of care, a key component in quality of care
Enhanced access (e.g., on-call, tele-triage)	Increased accessibility of care, a component of quality of care, through augmented provider availability to decrease use of ERs, walk-in clinics
Multidisciplinary teams (e.g., nurse practitioners)	Increased preventive care and health promotion counselling from nurse practitioners; redistribution of workload allows physicians to concentrate attention where skills are most needed
Enhanced information technology	Enhances coordination of care between multiple providers; reduces chance of medical error
Non-fee-for-service physician payment (e.g., capitation plus targeted bonuses)	Decreased volume incentives will lead to more appropriate care delivery

basic health and related information about the patient; a relationship with the patient that extends over time; a patient-provider relationship that incorporates mutual trust and personal regard; and, finally, a commitment on the part of the provider to collaborate with the patient in the management and coordination of diverse care services (14,15).

That continuity is linked to increased quality of care and enhanced outcomes appears certain from the existing literature. It has been shown to be associated with improved management of specific clinical conditions, such as diabetes (16), with enhanced preventive care (17), including childhood immunization (18), and with enhanced likelihood of patients complying with suggested treatments (19). Continuity is associated with higher patient satisfaction with care (20), itself an important component of quality of care. Finally, patients whose primary care incorporates continuity have lower rates of hospitalization (21,22) and make less frequent use of emergency departments (23).

Will the rostering which is central to proposals for primary care reform be likely to enhance continuity and thus to improve quality of care? It is difficult to imagine that rostering, *in itself*, will make any significant difference to the continuity of clinical care. Most patients currently think of themselves as affiliated with a specific family physician to which rostering would be simply an administrative addendum. In the absence of restrictions on patients or financial penalties to physicians for patients who seek service elsewhere, such as the capitation negation regulations that have been used in Ontario's Health Service Organizations, there are no incentives to provide continuity of service to rostered patients in a manner that differs from the current fee-for-service system. Moreover, since reformed primary care is built on group practice and a team approach to care, it is probable that patients will actually have a somewhat reduced chance of seeing their own physician compared to patients whose doctors remain in traditional solo practice.

ENHANCED ACCESS

Due to limited office hours and inadequate provision of on-call services it is said that primary care currently forces patients to use walk-in and after-hours clinics or, often for inappropriate concerns, emergency departments. Primary care reform is designed to enhance access to family physicians by mandating extended hours of clinic operation and augmented out-of-hours service, particularly the use of telephone triage by practice nurses. Is there evidence that such interventions will enhance clinical care?

A recent systematic review of models of after-hour primary care reached several conclusions about nurse telephone triage (24). It appears to effectively divert immediate care from physicians but in general does not reduce emergency room use or hospitalization rates. While the quality of advice has been found by a number of studies to be variable, serious medical misadventures do not appear associated with this form of care. Finally, patient satisfaction with telephone advice is generally low. Additional studies not captured in the review reinforce several of these points (25–27), suggesting that the clinical effectiveness and appropriateness of tele-triage as a first line of encounter in after-hours primary care has yet to be established.

The other important tactic of primary care reform for enhancing access is extended evening and weekend hours of clinic operation. This is intended to provide patients with an alternative to the use of both walk-in or after-hours clinics and emergency rooms. The assumption is that care from the patient's regular practice will enhance continuity and thereby increase quality. Unfortunately, current research evidence does not provide unequivocal support for this assumption.

In addition to emergency departments, service beyond regular office hours in Ontario can be obtained from walk-in clinics, group family practices, mixed clinics, and after-hours clinics. The distinctions amongst the first three organizations are often blurred since some walk-in clinics provide preventive care and service regular patients; however, after-hours clinics tend to provide strictly episodic care for acute illnesses (28). In 1991, walk-in clinics accounted for approximately 3 percent of the cost of initial patient visits and after-hours clinics about 2 percent (29). Patients are primarily motivated to use such facilities by convenience of time or location (30,31). However, in an Alberta study 43 percent of walk-in clinic patients sought service during times when the offices of their regular family physicians were open (32), suggesting that additional patient preferences may be at play.

Quality of care in a sample of Ontario walk-in clinics, family practices, and emergency departments was assessed for eight sentinel conditions. The scores for walk-in clinics and emergency departments were significantly higher than for family practices. As well, patient satisfaction, itself an important component of quality of care, has been shown to be higher for walk-in clinic than emergency department patients; only in respect to waiting times were family practice patients significantly more satisfied than persons attending walk-in clinics (33). Finally, surveyed walk-in clinic physicians, when compared to office-based family physicians, were less satisfied with relationships with patients, but more satisfied with availability of consultations, support staff, income, and vacation coverage (34). Importantly, physician employment satisfaction has been shown to be associated with the quality of care provided (35).

It is difficult to see from the evidence available to date how substituting tele-triage and extended office hours is likely to result in a substantial improvement in the quality of clinical care available to Ontario residents. Continuity will be enhanced, but possibly at the cost of patient preference and quality of the clinical care provided. A case can certainly be made for diverting trivial care from emergency rooms (36), but the justification here is more economic than clinical.

MULTIDISCIPLINARY TEAMS

A team approach to the provision of primary care is a common theme in current proposals for change. While many types of providers — social workers, pharmacists, psychologists, physiotherapists — are frequently mentioned, the one professional common to all discussions is that of nurse practitioner. In Ontario, the College of Nurses designation of "Primary Health Care Nurse Practitioner" equips the individual to provide comprehensive health services encompassing health promotion, prevention of diseases and injuries, cure, rehabilitation, and support services. The credential requires one year of additional training beyond a bachelor of nursing degree or two years beyond a nursing diploma. It is generally combined with the Extended Class designation which allows nurses to communicate a diagnosis, order diagnostic ultrasound and some x-rays, prescribe a defined range of drugs, and complete death certificates (37).

Compelling clinical evidence that nurse practitioners can play a significant role in the delivery of quality primary care dates from a landmark Canadian study published in 1974 (38). A randomized trial of the use of nurse practitioners compared to family physicians in Burlington, Ontario, found that patients in both care groups had similar mortality rates and no differences were found in physical capacity, social function, or emotional function. Quality of care was deemed similar and satisfaction among patients in both groups was high.

Substantial evidence has accumulated from various developed countries confirming the conclusions of the McMaster investigators. This literature was summarized in a systematic review in 2002. The authors identified 11 randomized trials and 23 observational studies comparing nurse practitioners and family doctors providing first-contact care to patients with undifferentiated health problems in a primary care setting. Patients were more satisfied with nurse practitioner care and no differences in patient health status were found. Though nurse practitioners tended to spend a longer time with patients and order more tests, no differences were found in the number of prescriptions, return visits or referrals to specialists (39).

To date the integration of nurse practitioners into the delivery of primary care has been tardy in Canada. This reticence is related to issues concerning funding, defining scope of practice boundaries, and practitioner concerns about liability; however, it cannot be attributed to a lack of evidence for the safety and effectiveness of nurse practitioners. While evidence supporting the effective integration of other types of providers into primary care delivery may be less developed, there is clearly a well-documented clinical rationale for family physician-nurse practitioner teams. Whether this evidence can be translated into effective team practice — that is, nurse practitioners functioning as complementary practitioners rather than doctor substitutes — remains to be established.

ENHANCED INFORMATION TECHNOLOGY

Information technology is held to be a significant component of primary care reform. Generally there are three types of clinical information functions: patient-specific information is generated on the care of patients and is referred to as the electronic medical record; knowledge-based systems provide information, such as clinical practice guidelines, to enhance patient care; and finally, decision support systems link patient data to knowledge sources to guide physicians in the management of clinical problems (40).

Hunt et al. performed a systematic review of the effect of computer-based decision support systems on physician performance and patient outcomes. Sixty-eight studies met the inclusion criteria. While relatively few studies addressed outcome, the authors drew several conclusions about decision support systems and physician behaviour: drug dosing was improved; preventive care was enhanced; and the management of a diverse group of medical conditions appeared to improve (41). Mitchell and Sullivan conducted a more recent systematic review of the impact of computer use during primary care appointments. Eighty-nine studies from the world literature met inclusion criteria. As in the study by Hunt et al., the authors noted a dearth of evidence on the effect on patient outcomes. However, they concluded that computer use did have an influence on several aspects of practice: the length of consultations increased; reminders for preventive care and some disease management situations appeared to improve the care process; there was increased prescribing of generic drugs; and fewer unnecessary tests were ordered (42).

These reviews present convincing evidence that information technology can enhance aspects of primary care delivery. In addition, it is worth noting that several Canadian studies illustrate that technology can also begin to address the lack of integration of primary care with other components of the health system. For example, when patients are discharged from a hospital a summary of their course while hospitalized is dictated by the attending physician and sent to the family physician to ensure continuity of care. Unfortunately, these discharge summaries are rarely received in a timely manner and often are uninformative on key points. A study of summaries on internal medicine patients discharged from two Ottawa teaching hospitals found that 34 percent lacked an admission diagnosis, 25 percent had no discharge diagnosis, and 23 percent did not include discharge medications. More disconcertingly, 40 percent were never received by the family physician (43). A subsequent randomized trial compared family physician impressions of a traditional dictated report with one generated from a database. The latter type of report was deemed to be as complete and informative as the traditional format (44). When these studies are coupled with findings from other jurisdictions that suggest that electronic discharge summaries can be available to family physicians within one hour of generation (45), the potential of information technology to greatly enhance the integration of primary care and the hospital sector is readily apparent. Such closer linkages, in turn, represent an important contribution to enhanced quality of care.

NON-FEE-FOR-SERVICE PHYSICIAN PAYMENT

For many practitioners the most radical — indeed, defining — component in primary care reform is the substitution of capitation payment for traditional fee-for-service remuneration. Unfortunately, there is a recognized paucity of reliable information on the relationship between physician remuneration methods and the quality of clinical care. We know that fee-for-service (FFS) promotes the delivery of more services (46) and that patients tend to prefer FFS in comparison to prepaid schemes (47–49). Two studies have found no short- or intermediate-term differences in health status outcomes for older patients when health maintenance organizations (HMO) are compared to FFS models (50,51). Similarly, studies focusing on individual clinical issues such as management of colorectal cancer (52), treatment of non-insulin dependent diabetes mellitus (53), or stroke survival (54) report no difference between HMO and FFS environments.

Some research attention has focused on the area of prevention. Little difference has been found in the United States between FFS and capitated practice in the provision of preventive care (55). In Ontario only modest differences were found between physicians paid by salary or capitation and those on FFS in terms of provision of preventive services (56). In contrast, in Quebec salaried physicians do appear to provide more preventive care than their FFS colleagues (57,58).

Relatively few attempts have been made to study payment method and quality in primary or ambulatory care settings. Two studies have examined process of care criteria, such as continuity, accessibility, or comprehensiveness, which are defining characteristics of primary care, in both instances finding FFS generally performed better than HMOs (59,60). Only two studies to date have examined the technical elements of clinical quality. Udvarhelyi et al. employed adequacy of blood pressure control and use of four screening procedures to evaluate clinical care, finding HMOs superior to FFS (61). Retchin and Brown used an expert panel to develop criteria concerning adequacy of history taking, physical examination, and use of screening procedures. A chart audit by trained nurse abstractors for 1590 Medicare patients found superior performance for HMOs (62).

A decade ago a paper from the Medical Outcomes Study in the United States stated: "We are unaware of any research that has attempted to comprehensively evaluate the quality of primary care delivered in prepaid and FFS systems" (59, p 1580). Five years later the authors of a review article found that: "There is no research on how changing payment methods in primary care affects the quality of care provided..." (63, p 16). A systematic review published in 2001 stated that while some aspects of physician behaviour appeared to change in response to alterations in funding method, "we are unable to make conclusions as to whether these changes are beneficial to patients" (64, p 53). Based on such sources it is clear that no clinical rationale yet exists in the research literature for a shift from fee-for-service to capitation payment.

CONCLUSION

How, then, can the evidence on the clinical rationale for primary care reform be assessed? One option might be to mimic loosely the method used by the Canadian Task Force on Preventive Health Care to weigh evidence for or against potential clinical activities (65). Based on such an approach, of the five key elements in primary care reform, rostered patients and non-fee-for-service payment are seen to be based on insufficient or conflicting evidence, enhanced access faces fair evidence against its adoption, enhanced information technology is supported by fair evidence, and the use of multidisciplinary teams has good evidence to support it (Table 3). These conclusions hardly provide a compelling evidentiary basis for policy-making.

There are, however, a number of limitations to such an approach. First, borrowing from the Canadian Task Force is largely arbitrary, since there is no universally agreed upon method of ranking evidence (66). Second, the systematic reviews upon which this study relies are a form of research originally intended as a method of synthesizing information on clinical interventions from numerous randomized controlled trials; however, the approach is much less reliable for assessing health service delivery issues where such trials are comparatively rare (67). Thirdly, by evaluating each of the components of primary care reform in isolation, it is possible that important beneficial synergies will be missed. Such synergies, however, remain speculative. Finally, it could be argued that the approach taken in this paper implies a naïve view of policy-making. That is, policy-makers seldom have the luxury of definitive evidence upon which to base decisions but, constrained by cost and public preferences, must simply choose options that have face credibility.

Despite such important caveats, however, it is difficult to detect a robust clinical rationale underlying current conceptions of primary care reform. The significant suspicion of reform initiatives on the part Ontario family physicians (68,69) may reflect an experiential wisdom that enhanced clinical outcomes are unlikely to result from the proposed changes. Unfortunately,

TABLE 3

KEY ELEMENTS, CLINICAL RATIONALE, AND ASSESSMENT OF EVIDENCE
OF PRIMARY CARE REFORM

Key Element	Clinical Rationale	Assessment of Evidence
Rostered patients	Closer doctor-patient relationship leading to enhanced continuity of care, itself a key component in quality of care	insufficient evidence to judge
Enhanced access (on-call, tele-triage)	Increased continuity of care through decreased use of ERs, walk-in clinics	fair evidence against
Multidisciplinary teams (nurse practitioners)	Increased preventive care and health promotion counselling from nurse practitioners; redistribution of work load allows physicians to concentrate attention where skills are most needed.	good evidence to support
Enhanced information technology	Enhances coordination of care between multiple providers; reduces chance of medical error.	fair evidence to support
Non-fee-for-service physician payment (capitation plus)	Decreased volume incentives will lead to more appropriate care delivery.	conflicting evidence; no conclusions

evaluations of pilot sites in the province are of little help in countering such skepticism (70,71). On balance, it seems fair to echo the conclusion of a recent overview of Canadian primary care policy:

> Discussions of innovations in primary care invariably take place in an evidentiary vacuum. Strong evidence is lacking to support the superiority of any one model of organizing, funding, and delivering primary care and of many suggested model components, including group practice, multidisciplinary practice, and remuneration methods. (72)

Seen in this light it appears questionable whether reformed primary care will bear the weight of the very substantial hopes pinned upon it by a sequence of provincial and national commissions.

REFERENCES

1   White KL, Williams F, Greenberg BG. The ecology of medical care. New England Journal of Medicine 1961;265:885–892.

2   Green LA, Fryer GE Jr., Yawn BP, Lanier D, Dovey SM. The ecology of medical care revisited. New England Journal of Medicine 2001;344:2021–2025.

3   Macinko J, Starfield B, Shi L. The contribution of primary care systems to health outcomes within Organisation for Economic Cooperation and Development (OECD) countries, 1970–1998. Health Services Research 2003;38(3):831–865.

4   Commission on the Future of Health Care in Canada. RJ Romanow, Commissioner. Building on values: the future of health care in Canada — final report. Ottawa: the Commission; 2002.

5   Canada. Parliament. Senate. Standing Committee on Social Affairs, Science and Technology. MJL Kirby, Chair. The health of Canadians — the federal role, final report on the state of the health care system in Canada. Ottawa: the Standing Committee; 2002.

6   New Brunswick. Health services review committee. Report of the Committee. Fredericton: Department of Health and Wellness; 1999.

7   Ontario. Health Services Restructuring Commission. Looking back, looking forward; the Ontario health services restructuring commission, 1996–2000: a legacy report. Toronto: the Commission; 2000.

8   Quebec. Study Commission on Health and Social Services. Emerging solutions: report and recommendations. Quebec: the Commission; 2000.

9   Alberta. Premier's Advisory Council on Health. D Mazankowski, Chair. Report of the Premier's Advisory Council on Health: a framework for reform. Edmonton: the Council; 2001.

10   Saskatchewan Commission on Medicare. KJ Fyke, Commissioner. Caring for medicare: sustaining a quality system. Regina: Policy and Planning Branch, Saskatchewan Health; 2001.

11   Canada. Health Canada. Primary Health Care Transition Fund. Available at http://www.hc-sc.gc.ca/phctf-fassp/english/index.html Accessed October 23, 2003.

12   Ontario. Ministry of Health and Long-Term Care. Primary care reform in Ontario. Available at http://www.health.gov.on.ca/english/public/updates/archives/hu_03/docnurse/pricare_fs.html Accessed October 23, 2003.

13   McWhinney I. Primary care: core values. Core values in a changing world. British Medical Journal 1998;316:1807–1809.

14   Saultz WJ. Defining and measuring interpersonal continuity of care. Annals of Family Medicine 2003;1(3):1340–1343.

15   Reid R, Haggerty J, McKendry R. Defusing the confusion: concepts and measures of continuity of health care. Vancouver: Centre for Health Services and Policy Research, University of British Columbia. Report. March 2002.

16   Parchman ML, Pugh JA, Noel PH, Larme AC. Continuity of care, self-management behaviors, and glucose control in patients with type 2 diabetes. Medical Care 2002;40(2):137–144.

17   Kasper JD. The importance of type of usual source of care for children's physician access and expenditures. Medical Care 1987;25:386–398.

18   Christakis DA, Mell L, Wright J, Davis R, Connell FA. The association between greater continuity of care and timely measles-mumps-rubella vaccination. American Journal of Public Health 2000;90:962–965.

19   Hjortdahl P, Laerum E. Continuity of care in general practice: effect on patient satisfaction. British Medical Journal 1992;304:1287–1290.

20   Nutting PA, Goodwin MA, Flocke SA, Zyzanski SJ, Stange KC. Continuity of primary care: to whom does it matter and when? Annals of Family Medicine 2003;1(3):149–155.

21   Gill JM, Mainous AG. The role of provider continuity in preventing hospitalizations. Archives of Family Medicine 1998;7:351–357.

22   Mainour AG, Gill JM. The importance of continuity of care in the likelihood of future hospitalization: is site of care equivalent to a primary clinician? American Journal of Public Health 1998;88:1539-1541.

23   Christakis DA, Mell L, Koepsell TD, Zummerman FJ, Connell FA. Association of lower continuity of care with greater risk of emergency department use and hospitalization in children. Pediatrics 2001;107:524–529.

24   Leibowitz R, Day S, Dunt D. A systematic review of the effect of different models of after-hours primary medical care services on clinical outcome, medical workload, and patient and GP satisfaction. Family Practice 2003;20(3):311–317.

25   Payne F, Shipman C, Dale J. Patients' experiences of receiving telephone advice from a GP co-operative. Family Practice 2001;18(2):156–160.

26   Lee TJ, Guzy J, Johnson D, Woo H, Baraff LJ. Caller satisfaction with after-hours telephone advice: nurse advice service versus on-call pediatricians. Pediatrics 2002;110(5): 865–872.

27   Lee TJ, Baraff LM, Guzy J, Johnson D, Woo H. Does telephone triage delay significant medical treatment? Advice nurse service vs on-call pediatricians. Archives of Pediatric Adolescent Medicine 2003;157:635–641.

28   Barnsley J, Williams AP, Kacaorowski J, Vayda E, Vingilis E, Campbell A, Atkin K. Who provides walk-in services? Survey of primary care practices in Ontario. Canadian Family Physician 2002;48:519–526.

29   Weinkauf DJ, Kralj B, Medical service provision and costs: do walk-in clinics differ from other primary care delivery settings? Canadian Public Policy/Analyse de Politiques 1998;24(4):471–484.

30   Jones M. Walk-in primary medical care centers: lessons from Canada. British Medical Journal 2000;321:928–931.

31   Brown JB, Sangster LM, Ostbye T, Barnsley JM, Mathews M, Ogilvie G. Walk-in clinics: patient expectations and family physician availability. Family Practice 2002;19(2):202–206.

32   Szafran O, Bell NR. Use of walk-in clinics by rural and urban patients. Canadian Family Physician 2000;46:114–119.

33   Hutchison B, Ostbye T, Barnsley J, Stewart M, Mathews M, Campbell MK, Vayda E, Harris SB, Torrance-Rynard V, Tyrrell C. Patient satisfaction and quality of care in walk-in clinics, family practices and emergency departments: the Ontario walk-in study. Canadian Medical Association Journal 2003;168(8):977–983.

34   Williams AP, Barnsley J, Vayda E, Kaczorowski J, Ostbye T, Wenghofer E. Comparing the characteristics and attitudes of physicians in different primary care settings: the Ontario Walk-in Study. Family Practice 2002;19(5):647–657.

35   Williams ES, Skinner AC. Outcomes of physician job satisfaction: a narrative review, implications, and directions for future research. Health Care Management Review 2003;28(2):119–140.

36   Burnett MG, Grover SA. Use of the emergency department for nonurgent care during regular business hours. Canadian Medical Association Journal 1996;154(9):1345-1351.

37   Dacres L, Clark B. A primer on nurse practitioners and RN (EC)s. Communique, Colleges of Nurses of Ontario 2003;28:6–7. Available at www.cno.org/publications/cmg/cmgvol28no1.pdf Accessed October 23, 2003.

38   Spitzer WO, Sackett DL, Sibley JC, Roberts RS, Tech M, Gent M, Kergin DJ, Hackett BC, Olynich A. The Burlington randomized trial of the nurse practitioner. New England Journal of Medicine 1974;290(5):251–256.

39   Horrocks S, Anderson E, Salisbury C. Systematic review of whether nurse practitioners working in primary care can provide equivalent care to doctors. British Medical Journal 2002;324:819–823.

40   Hersh WR. Medical informatics. Journal of the American Medical Association 2002;288(16):1955–1958.

41   Hunt DL, Haynes RB, Hanna SE, Smith K. Effects of computer-based clinical decision support systems on physician performance and patient outcomes. Journal of the American Medical Association 1998;280(15):1339–1346,

42   Mitchell E, Sullivan F. A descriptive feast but an evaluative famine: systematic review of published articles on primary care computing during 1980–97. British Medical Journal 2001;322(7281):279–282.

43   van Walraven C, Weinberg AL. Quality assessment of a discharge summary system. Canadian Medical Association Journal 1995;152(9):1437–1442.

44   van Walraven C, Laupacis A, Seth R, Wells G. Dictated versus database-generated discharge summaries: a randomized clinical trial. Canadian Medical Association Journal 1999;160(3):319–326.

45   Branger PJ, van der Wouden JC, Schudel BR, Verboog E, Duisterhout JS, van der Lei J, van Bemmel JH. Electronic communication between providers of primary and secondary care. British Medical Journal 1992;305(6861):1068–1070.

46   Shimmura K. Effects of different remuneration methods on general medical practice: a comparison of capitation and fee-for-service payment. International Journal of Health Planning Management 1988;3:245–258.

47   Davies AR, Ware JE Jr, Brook RH, Peterson JR, Newhouse JP. Consumer acceptance of prepaid and fee-for-service medical care: results from a randomized controlled trial. Health Services Research 1986;21(3):429–452.

48   Murray JP. A follow-up comparison of patient satisfaction among prepaid and fee-for-service patients. Journal of Family Practice 1988;26(5):576–681.

49   Rubin HR, Gandek B, Rogers WH, Kosinski M, McHorney CA, Ware JE. Patients' ratings of outpatient visits in different practice settings. Journal of the American Medical Association 1993;270(7):835–840.

50   Lurie N, Christianson J, Finch M, Moscovice I. The effects of capitation on health and functional status of the medicaid elderly. A randomized trial. Annals of Internal Medicine 1994;120(6):506–511.

51   Ware JE, Bayliss MS, Rogers WH, Kosinski M, Tarlow AR. Differences in 4-year health outcomes for elderly and poor, chronically ill patients treated in HMO and fee-for-service systems. Journal of the American Medical Association 1996;276(13):1039–1047.

52   Vernon SW, Hughes JI, Heckel VM, Jackson GL. Quality of care for colorectal cancer in a fee-for-service and health maintenance organization practice. Cancer 1992;69(10):2418–2425.

53   Greenfield S, Rogers W, Mangotich M, Carney MF, Tarlov AR. Outcomes of patients with hypertension and non-insulin-dependent diabetes mellitus treated by different systems and specialties. Journal of the American Medical Association 1995;274(18):1436–1444.

54   Retchin SM, Brown RS, Yeh SC, Chu D, Moreno L. Outcomes of stroke patients in medicare fee for service and managed care. Journal of the American Medical Association 1997;278(2):119–124.

55   Ellsbury KE, Montano DE, Parker JJ. Preventive services in a hybrid capitation and fee-for-service setting. Journal of Family Practice 1988;28:540–544.

56   Hutchison B, Woodward C, Norman G, Abelson J, Brown J. Provision of preventive care to unannounced standardized patients: correlates of evidence-based practice. Hamilton, ON: McMaster University Centre for Health Economics and Policy Analysis, Working Paper Series 97-94;1997.

57   Battista RN, Spitzer WO. Adult cancer prevention in primary care: contrasts among primary care practice settings in Quebec. American Journal of Public Health 1983;73:1040–1041.

58   Battista RN, Williams JI, MacFarlane LA. Determinants of primary medical practice in adult cancer prevention. Medical Care 1986;24:216–224.

59   Safran DG, Tarlov AR, Rogers WH. Primary care performance in fee-for-service and prepaid health care systems. Journal of the American Medical Association 1994;271(20):1579–1586.

60   Safran DG, Wilson IB, Rogers WH, Montgomery JE, Chang H. Primary care quality in the medicare program. Comparing the performance of medicare health maintenance organizations and traditional fee-for-service medicare. Archives of Internal Medicine 2002;162:757–765.

61   Udvarhelyi IS, Jennison K, Phillips RS, Epstein AM. Comparison of the quality of ambulatory care for fee-for-service and prepaid patients. Annals of Internal Medicine 1991;115(5):394–400.

62   Retchin SM, Brown B. The quality of ambulatory care in medicare health maintenance organizations. American Journal of Public Health 1990;80(4):411–415.

63   Cumming J, Mays N. Shifting to capitation in primary care: what might the impact be in New Zealand? Australian Health Review 1999;22:8–24.

64   Gosden T, Forland F, Kristiansen IS, Sutton M, Leese B, Giuffrida A, Sergison M, Pedersen L. Impact of payment method on behaviour of primary care physicians: a systematic review. Journal of Health Services and Research Policy 2001;6(1):44

65   Canadian Task Force on Preventive Health Care, History/Methodology, available at http://www.ctfphc.org/ Accessed October 23, 2003.

66   Upshur REG. Are all evidence-based practices alike? Problems in the ranking of evidence. Canadian Medical Association Journal 2003;169(7):677–680.

67   Petticrew M. Why certain systematic reviews reach uncertain conclusions. British Medical Journal 2003;326:756–758.

68   Neimanis IM, Paterson JM, Allega RL. Physicians' participation in Hamilton-Wentworth. Canadian Family Physician 2002;48:306–313.

69   Cohen M, Ferrier B, Woodward CA, Brown J. Health Care system reform: Ontario family physicians' reactions. Canadian Family Physician 2001;47:1777–1784.

70   Ontario. Ministry of Health and Long-Term Care. Evaluation of Primary Care Reform Pilots in Ontario Phase I. Final report. Toronto: the Ministry; 2001.

71   Ontario. Ministry of Health and Long-Term Care. Evaluation of Primary Care Reform Pilots in Ontario Phase 2. Interim report. Toronto: the Ministry; 2001.

72   Hutchison B, Abelson J, Lavis J. Primary care in Canada: so much innovation, so little change. Health Affairs 2001;20(3):116–31.

Rationales for Primary Health Care Reform: Why Are We Doing This?

An Economic Perspective

Raisa Deber

Primary care reform is a complex concept, interpreted in a variety of ways (1,2). Other papers in this volume deal with various of its potential features, including continuity of care, 24/7 access, and health teams. This paper will concentrate on the implications of one frequently proposed model — moving from paying clinicians on the basis of fee-for-service to a set (capitated) fee for each member of the defined (rostered) population for which they are clinically responsible. It suggests that insistence on capitated funding may, in turn, undermine many of the other goals of primary care reform.

The economic view of the world carries with it a number of basic assumptions. As applied to primary care reform, it assumes that how you pay people contains incentives to do (or not do) particular things. From this, it follows that changing how people are paid is likely to change these incentives. Incentives may encourage them to do more, less, or to do different things. Economists accordingly speak of the need to "align incentives" and ensure that the incentives inherent in the payment scheme encourage the behaviour needed to achieve desired policy goals.

It must be recognized that health professionals, with a clear code of ethics, often do not behave as economic maximizers. For example, an alternative payment plan in an Ontario medical school was found to have no impact on either the number or the variety of surgical procedures provided to patients (3). It nonetheless appears unwise to set up mechanisms with hopes that providers will act against their own economic self-interest, but reserve the highest financial rewards for those least willing to abide by such professionally induced constraints.

The primary mechanisms for paying physicians are fee-for-service, capitation, and salary. Because no single individual can provide 24/7 care, capitation-based payment also requires a shift from solo practice to a "provider organization" which has the resources to provide the agreed-upon scope of services outside of office hours. Capitation is thus in part an incentive to change how care is organized. The organization receiving capitation payments may in turn purchase services from providers in a number of ways (including as simple a mechanism as continuing with business as usual during office hours, but contracting out after-hours care to another organization). Thus, capitation payments to an organization do not require that the individuals actually providing services also be paid by capitation; they may be paid for their time (e.g., via a salary or sessional fees) and/or for the particular services they provide.

In his comprehensive review of the advantages and disadvantages of these payment mechanisms, Robinson notes that none are perfect; all contain inappropriate incentives.

> Fee-for-service rewards the provision of inappropriate services, the fraudulent upcoding of visits and procedures, and the churning of "ping-pong" referrals among specialists. Capitation rewards the denial of appropriate services, the dumping of the chronically ill, and a narrow scope of practice that refers out every time-consuming patient. Salary undermines productivity, condones on-the-job leisure, and fosters a bureaucratic mentality in which every procedure is someone else's problem (4, p 149)

Robinson accordingly suggests paying greater attention both to blended payment mechanisms, and the host of non-price mechanisms by which appropriate behaviour can be monitored and motivated. A similar analysis, within the context of promoting shared mental health care in Canada, reached similar conclusions (5).

Capitation payments have a number of characteristics. First, in contrast to fee-for-service, payment is prospective, and the sum available per patient is capped. A logical response by providers to capped payments is to try to control their cost structures. In theory, this gives providers incentives to be efficient in their provision of services, and should lead to less variability in professional practice as each adopts "best practices." However, it may also carry incentives to offload care to organizations outside the capitated practice. For example, in a letter to *Canadian Family Physician*, a Glasgow-trained family doctor suggested that, under capitation, "we were encouraged to enrol as many patients as possible to maximize our income but were discouraged from treating them." Instead, as much care as possible was referred to the local hospital, whose costs were not charged back to the practice (6).

In the United States, payment has been shifting away from fee-for-service payment to capitation, with health maintenance organizations receiving fixed payments to provide health care, and often contracting with other providers to provide these services on a capitation basis (7).

However, costs may be incurred as a result of factors beyond the control of providers. Certain patients have more severe underlying conditions, and need more time and services (8). Treating such patients exposes providers to extra costs, and lowers their net incomes. The usual response by advocates of capitation has been attempts to "risk adjust" the payment rates. While in theory this should be effective; in practice, existing risk adjustment methods are relatively ineffective (9). They often account for only a modest percentage of the variation in costs. Incomplete risk adjustment results in payments that are too high for some providers and too low for others. Over time, underpaid providers either exit the market or begin to systematically avoid high-cost patients, while overpaid providers remain in the market and continue to reap undeserved rewards (4).

CAPITATION: SETTING THE FORMULA

From a system-wide perspective, setting a per capita payment allows predictability of expenditures. If costs rise beyond the level envisioned in the payments (whether through new therapies or inflation in labour costs or higher prices paid for goods), the risk of these higher costs are transferred away from payers, and assumed by both providers (for the services included in the basket) and patients (for those which are not). We consider three potential problems which providers must consider: (i) cost structures, (ii) volatility and (iii) cream skimming.

Cost Structures

Health providers can be viewed as "firms," which convert such resources as labour (time and skills), raw materials, and plant and equipment into a product (10). For a given set of inputs, there will be a maximum amount of product which can be produced. Economists can express these relationships in production functions and cost functions. An efficient firm will produce goods at the minimum unit cost. The input resources, in turn, are divided into fixed costs (capital, plant, and equipment), and the variable costs needed to produce each additional unit of output. In the long run, there are no fixed costs; firms can chose to expand or contract to alter constraints on their capacity. Nonetheless, these costs can be "lumpy" — that is, one usually cannot hire one hour of a physician, nurse, or nutritionist to manage a temporary bottleneck. In general, revenues tend to be less lumpy — firms will receive a reimbursement for each unit they sell.

Most practices have high fixed costs for such items as maintaining an office (rent, heat, telephone, equipment) and staffing it. The marginal cost of seeing one more patient, assuming the infrastructure can absorb it, is probably small. The problem arises when the cost side is lumpy while the revenues are not. Capitation formulas are usually based on a notion of the average costs of handling the rostered patients. If the cost structure is lumpy, then adding an additional patient, at the margin, will generate a "surplus" (in that the additional payment will be greater than the cost of handling him/her), while losing a patient, at the margin, will generate a "deficit" (in that the payment loss is greater than the "savings" from not seeing him/her). Similar problems can arise in other sectors with lumpy cost structures, such as school boards, hospitals, or universities, if they are paid on an average-cost basis. Under those circumstances, if the cost of having an additional student in a class (or patient on an under-capacity ward) is trivial, the fiscal gain can be substantial. Conversely, if savings from having one less student, or one less patient, are trivial (i.e., the class, or ward, must still be staffed), the fiscal loss from enrollment decline can pose a major threat to sustainability for those students or patients remaining.

In the case of physicians, overheads have been estimated at 28 to 36 percent of gross income (11). Although detailed breakdowns of these costs into rent, staff, and supplies are not readily available, it seems likely that physician offices have lumpy cost structures, which may not fit well with capitated formulas. It would seem relatively simple to ensure that funding formulas be blended to take proper account of cost structures and avoid having windfall gains, or losses, arise from small changes in practice sizes. The Quebec model, discussed in this volume, is a good example of a formula that begins with the actual costs of running a practice, as opposed to basing this on average costs.

However, even assuming the payment is (on average) sufficient to cover average costs, capitation may still present fiscal risks for providers.

Volatility

Volatility arises because averages are just that; peaks and valleys occur. Capitated models assume that providers will receive a sum sufficient to cover the utilization (claims) of the individuals they cover. In effect, they receive an average, which can be seen as covering the cost of a randomly selected person in that pool. However, to the extent that the distribution of expenditures does not group tightly around its mean, payments will be too generous for those falling below the mean and inadequate for those in the upper tail. The statistical laws of large numbers imply that these issues will be particularly problematic at smaller units of aggregation. The smaller the unit, the more difficult it is to spread these risks, both over time and over clients. One very high cost client can thus lead to bankruptcy. A tension can thus arise between stability and integration. Primary care reform often talks about care integration, and the desire to have a comprehensive array of services in the "primary care package" to improve coordination. However, adding more services gives problems, both in terms of critical mass (will small practices have the expertise?), but also in terms of increased volatility, and the associated fiscal risk. For example, a recent policy synthesis suggested that "funding of primary care should be allowed on a per capita formula and should include specialized medical and hospital services, drugs, diagnostic and therapeutic services, homecare and palliative services" (1). Regardless of its merits in promoting clinical integration, this model runs the risk of introducing a high degree of volatility and fiscal risk. If one wishes to base primary care reform on units with a relatively small number of patients, it is probably unwise to make them fiscally responsible for such a wide scope of services. If variation is random, then such volatility is likely to even out over time; high spending years might be followed by low spending ones. Such circumstances could be managed through some combination of large enough groups (Primary Care Groups in the United Kingdom average 100,000 clients [12]), and reinsurance/stop-loss protection against catastrophic expenditures.

Cream Skimming

However, these solutions will be less effective if variation is not random. Who wins and who loses will depend upon the relationship between the distribution of actual expenditures and the results of each funding formula. Providers can profit if they can systematically select those individuals likely to be most profitable (which usually implies that they have better information than do the payers setting the capitation payments). This term is often referred to as "risk selection" or by such food analogies as "cream skimming" (although in Germany, it is sometimes called "picking the raisins"). Depending upon who is doing the selection, and how much control individuals have over whether these adverse events are likely to occur, economists often use the term "adverse selection."

For capitated payment systems, the most profitable patients tend to be those at lowest risk, and there are incentives to avoid high cost individuals. A variety of studies have clarified that providers indeed are influenced by these incentives. For example, a study of a managed care program for blind and disabled beneficiaries in Tennessee found "substantial evidence of persistent risk selection among plans" (13). An American study found that 40 percent of the physicians they surveyed "encouraged more complex and ill patients to avoid capitated plans" and 23 percent encouraged their healthier patients to join (14).

In theory, good information can ensure that such risk selection cannot happen. With appropriate information, budgetary allocations could be "risk adjusted" to ensure that the categories are more homogeneous. Considerable attention has been paid to this question, and a number of methods have been developed. They are seen as particularly high priority in systems without single payers (e.g., the US, Germany, and the Netherlands), but are also receiving attention in the UK and Canada. Primary care physicians are paid by capitation in many jurisdictions, although these usually co-exist with salary or fee-for-service components (12). However, several reviews of risk adjustment have reached similar conclusions: there is no commonly accepted way of doing risk adjustment, and existing approaches do not explain much of the variation in expenditures (7,12,15–18).

Some of the proposed systems for risk adjustment require extensive information, and are considered expensive and unwieldy to implement. For example, a UK review notes that a system developed by Johns Hopkins generates up to 32 aggregated diagnostic groups per person, and then places patients into one of around 100 mutually exclusive "adjusted clinical groups" (7). Administrative costs to capture this amount of data can be high. Even so, these systems are known to be poor at dealing with outlier cases; they are also vulnerable to providers "upcoding" by tweaking the recorded codes in order to classify patients into groups attracting higher payments (16).

In practice, most risk adjustment methods focus on age and sex alone. Although in theory, additional factors (e.g., case mix, morbidity) could be added, they rarely are. None of the risk adjustment models have predicted more than 10 percent of the variance in health care costs; those using primarily age and sex account for 1 to 3 percent of the variance (12,15).

The potential impact of differential risk depends in large part on the distribution of health expenditures. If the variation is minimal, then gains (or losses) would be constrained. If spending is skewed, however, the implications can be considerable. In the US, 10 percent of Medicaid enrollees were found to account for around 70 percent of all Medicaid payments (19).

Forget, Deber and Roos examined actual expenditures for individually attributable physician and hospital services — the services which must be publicly insured under the terms of the *Canada Health Act* — in the Canadian province of Manitoba between 1997 and 1999 (20–22). Health expenditures were found to be heavily skewed. The healthiest 50 percent of Manitobans used about 4 percent of resources, while the sickest 1 percent used 26 percent. In every age group, at least 80 percent of all people incurred costs less than the average for that age, while a small proportion incurred very high expenditures. Their results paralleled those found in an analysis of the US National Medical Expenditure Studies (23). For this paper, we analyzed costs for physician services only.

MANITOBA DATA

The Manitoba Population Health Research Data Repository, which is managed by the Manitoba Centre for Health Policy, captures standardized data, based on almost every physician and hospital contact in Manitoba (24). This information is anonymized, and all uses are subject to approval from Manitoba Health. The validity, reliability and usefulness of the data have been established through several previous studies (24,25) and are recognized as a unique resource for policy-makers (26,27). The data for Manitoba are broadly representative of Canada. Although the province represents about 4 percent of the Canadian population, it typically ranks in the middle with respect to major socioeconomic and demographic variables. In collaboration with the Manitoba Centre, we analyzed physician expenditures. We first assigned costs to individuals and then ordered the population into deciles based on their annual expenditure. If utilization were evenly distributed across the population, then the lowest spending 10 percent would be incurring approximately 10 percent of the cost, and so on.

Figure 1 shows the Lorenz curve for total physician and hospital costs, using 1997-99 averages. The Lorenz curve plots the cumulative proportion of ordered individuals against the cumulative proportion of expenditures. If there is no inequality, the Lorenz curve forms a straight diagonal line, called the line of equality.

Figure 2 shows a similar Lorenz curve for 1999 expenditures for physician services. These amounted to an average of $253 per capita; however, the lowest spending ("healthiest"?) 80 percent of Manitobans accounted for 12.44 percent of expenditures on physician fees. Even taking a three-year average (1997-99), they accounted for 18.21 percent of expenditures. This is noteworthy, since Ontario has announced its intention to have 80 percent of the province's

32   *Raisa Deber*

FIGURE 1

LORENZ CURVE FOR TOTAL COSTS (HOSPITAL + PHYSICIAN), MANITOBA: FISCAL 1997-1999

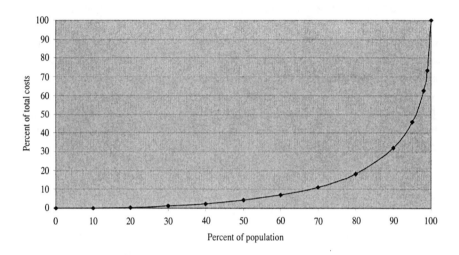

FIGURE 2

LORENZ CURVE FOR PHYSICIAN FEES, MANITOBA: FISCAL 1999

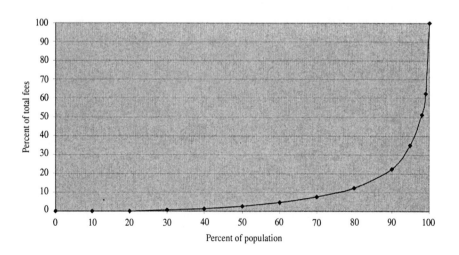

residents covered by reformed primary care models. In the hypothetical event that government decides to pay providers based on population spending, and directs 80 percent of the payments for physician services to cover 80 percent of the population, providers who can identify high cost individuals and omit them from a roster will be rewarded financially. If they can select the healthiest 80 percent, they will be receiving 80 percent of the money to defray about 18 percent of the costs, while those who agree to take the high cost patients will lose money. This hardly seems a good prescription for cost control.

What if payments were controlled for age? Figure 3 shows that average physician expenditure does indeed vary by age group. However, the skewness remains within each age group. Figure 4 shows the distribution for those age 20-24; the mean payment is $206.58, but it is heavily skewed. Indeed, figure 5 shows that this skewing remains even within the highest decile. Figure 6 shows that the same pattern applies for those age 75+, where the mean spending is $689.11. Figure 7 demonstrates the same pattern for those age 45-64, where the mean is $341.30. Indeed, the same pattern holds in *every* age-sex group; 80-90 percent of the population spends less than the mean of that group for physician plus hospital services, and about 70-80 percent spends less than the mean for physician services alone.

FIGURE 3

MEAN PHYSICIAN COSTS, MANITOBA 1999, BY AGE GROUP

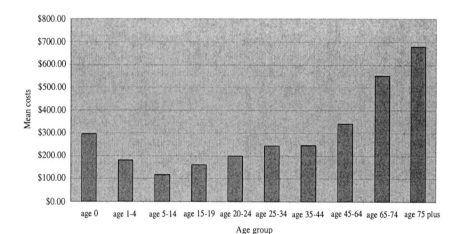

FIGURE 4

MEAN PHYSICIAN FEES, MANITOBA 1999, BY DECILE (AGE 20-24)

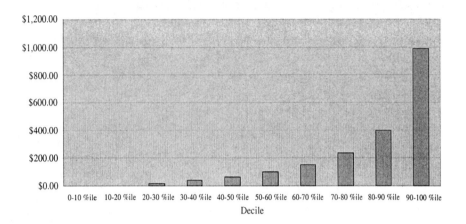

FIGURE 5

MEAN PHYSICIAN EXPENDITURES, HIGHEST DECILE, MANITOBA 1999
(AGE 20-24)

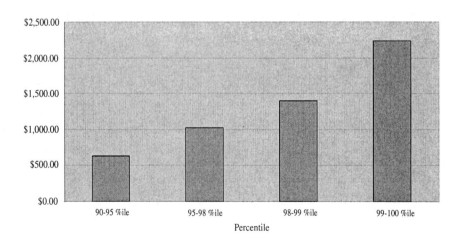

FIGURE 6
MEAN PHYSICIAN FEES, MANITOBA 1999, BY DECILE (AGE 75+)

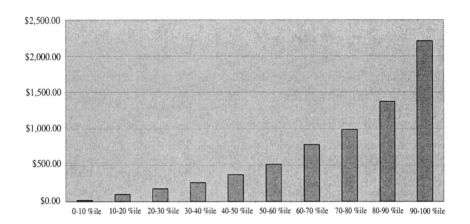

FIGURE 7
MEAN PHYSICIAN FEES, MANITOBA 1999, BY DECILE (AGE 45-64)

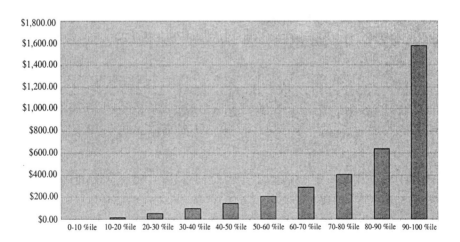

CONCLUSIONS

Canadian doctors have been debating the place of capitation vs. fee-for-service (6,28–30). Not surprisingly, they are not attracted to a model whose key purpose is the shifting of financial risk for additional utilization from government to physicians. The relatively slow response of Canadian physicians to proposed primary care reform models also suggests that capitation is likely to attract considerable opposition. Coupled with suggestions that such models may undermine provision of care to the most vulnerable populations, one is left with the question of the goal of primary care reform. If the purpose is largely clinical, with such aims as improving coordination, quality, and appropriateness, then capitation does not seem to be an essential element of primary care reform. Recognizing the limitations of fee-for-service, other blended models may be preferable. Indeed, although a study of 13 industrialized countries found that a strong primary care infrastructure was an important determinant of health, capitated funding was not among the key characteristics which distinguished those countries with good overall health from those with poorer outcomes (31).

Because health spending is so heavily skewed, simple capitation formulae give precisely the wrong incentives to providers and discourage enrollment of the sickest. On clinical grounds, the sickest may be most likely to benefit from continuity of care and the other goals of primary care reform. In the unlikely event that capitation is forced on providers, most will probably continue to try to give the best care to their patients. Those who do, however, are most likely to be penalized by poorly conceived funding formulae, which seems less than wise. It appears inappropriate to reward cream skimming and penalize good care for high needs populations. If the policy goals are restricted to financial predictability and shifting risks to providers and patients, capitation may indeed succeed, but it would seem that there are other ways of accomplishing those goals which would be less clinically disruptive.

ACKNOWLEDGMENTS

This project is funded from a grant by CIHR. Sincere thanks to my co-researchers Leslie Roos, Evelyn Forget, and Randy Walld, and to Heather Chappel and the M-THAC Research Unit.

REFERENCES

1   Lamarche PA, Beaulieu M-D, Pineault R, Contandriopoulos A-P, Denis J-L, Haggerty J. Choices for change: the path for restructuring primary healthcare services in Canada.

Final report. Ottawa: Canadian Health Services Research Foundation; 2003. Available at http://www.chsrf.ca/search_e.php

2   Starfield B. Primary care: balancing health needs, services and technology. New York: Oxford University Press; 1998.

3   Shortt SED, Stanton S. Does changing the way doctors are paid change the way they practice? Evidence from an Ontario Academic Health Science Centre. Ottawa: Canadian Health Services Research Foundation Paper, June, 2001.

4   Robinson JC. Theory and practice in the design of physician payment incentives. Milbank Quarterly 2001;79(2):149–177.

5   Dewa CS, Hoch JS, Goering P. Using financial incentives to promote shared mental health care. Canadian Journal of Psychiatry 2001;46:488–495.

6   Draper L. Choosing fee-for-service. Canadian Family Physician 2002;48:1612.

7   Majeed A, Bindman AB, Weiner JP. Use of risk adjustment in setting budgets and measuring performance in primary care I: how it works. British Medical Journal 2001;323:604–607.

8   Newhouse JP. Health reform in the United States. Economic Journal 1996;106:1713–24.

9   Newhouse JP. Risk adjustment: where are we now? Inquiry 1998;35:122–131.

10 Evans RG. Strained mercy: the economics of Canadian health care. Toronto: Butterworths & Co.; 1984.

11 Buske L. Net earnings for FPs, specialists. Canadian Medical Association Journal 2002;167(5):535.

12 Hutchison B, Hurley J, Reid R, et al. Capitation formulae for integrated health systems: a policy synthesis. Ottawa: Canadian Health Services Research Foundation; 1999.

13 Hill SC, Thornton C, Trenholm C, Wooldridge J. Risk selection among SSI enrollees in TennCare. Inquiry 2002;39(2):152–167.

14 Wynia MK, Zucker D, Supran S, Selker HP. Patient protection and risk selection: do primary care physicians encourage their patients to join or avoid capitated health plans according to the patients' health status? Journal of General Internal Medicine 2002;17(1):40–47.

15 Hurley J, Hutchison B, Giacomini M et al. Policy considerations in implementing capitation for integrated health systems: a policy synthesis. Ottawa: Canadian Health Services Research Foundation Document Series; 1999.

16 Majeed A, Bindman AB, Weiner JP. Use of risk adjustment in setting budgets and measuring performance in primary care II: advantages, disadvantages, and practicalities. British Medical Journal 2001;323:607–610.

17 Scheffler RM. Adverse selection: the achilles heel of the NHS reforms. Lancet 1989;1(8644):950–952.

18 Giacomini M, Luft HS, Robinson JC. Risk adjusting community-rated health plan premiums: a survey of risk assessment literature and policy applications. Annual Review of Public Health 1995;16:401–430.

19 US Department of Health and Human Services. Medicare and Medicaid statistical supplement. Health Care Financial Review 1996;17(Suppl):1.

20 Forget EL, Deber RB, Roos LL. Medical savings accounts: will they reduce costs? Canadian Medical Association Journal 2002;167(2):143–147.

21 Deber RB, Forget E, Roos LL, Walld R. Medical savings accounts in a universal system: wishful thinking meets evidence. Health Policy 2004;in press.

22 Forget E, Deber RB, Roos LL, Walld R. Recent market-based challenges to Canada's scheme: a gender analysis. Feminist Economics 2004;in press.

23   Berk ML, Monheit AC. The concentration of health care expenditures, revisited. Health Affairs 2001;20(2):9–18.

24   Roos LL Jr, Mustard CA, Nicol JP et al. Registries and administrative data: organization and accuracy. Medical Care 1993;31(3):201–212.

25   Roos LL, Nicol JP. A research registry: uses, development, and accuracy. Journal of Clinical Epidemiology 1999;52(1):39–47.

26   Roos NP, Black C, Frohlich N et al. Population health and health care use: an information system for policy makers. Milbank Quarterly 1996;74(1):3–31.

27   Roos LL, Roos NP. Of space and time, of health care and health. Journal of Health Services Research and Policy 2001;6(2):120–122.

28   Rosser WW, Kasperski J. Argument for blended funding. Canadian Family Physician 2002;48:247–249.

29   Mulligan PK. Capitation: the wrong direction for primary care reform. Canadian Family Physician 2002;48:233–235.

30   Mulligan PK. Capitation by any other name. Canadian Family Physician 2002;48:258.

31   Starfield B, Shi L. Policy relevant determinants of health: an international perspective. Health Policy 2002;60(3):201–218.

Experience Abroad I
Primary Care Reform in the UK

Bonnie Sibbald, Rod Sheaff and Martin Roland

THE NATURE OF PRIMARY CARE REFORM

The National Health Service (NHS) of the UK is funded from taxation and free at the point of delivery. Its goal is to deliver health care which is effective, efficient and equitable. There is uncertainty as to what model of health care organization might best fulfil these goals, and the past 20 years have seen unremitting reform as successive governments have experimented with new approaches. Broadly speaking, the NHS has moved from a *hierarchical* model of care delivery in the 1980s to a *quasi-market* in the 1990s, and then to a *network* in the twenty-first century.

Hierarchy

The NHS of the 1980s could be characterized as a hierarchical "command and control" system with policy and practice determined centrally by the government and implemented through local health care organizations that were accountable to government for their performance. All health care organizations, apart from general practice, were directly owned and operated through this hierarchy. General practice was, and is, distinctive in that general practitioners (GPs) are not directly employed by the NHS but provide services to the NHS under a nationally negotiated contract. Local health care organizations administered the GP contract on behalf of government but had virtually no power to shape general practice provision to meet local needs.

The system provided few incentives to modernize, improve efficiency, or respond to user demands. It was overly bureaucratic, slow to adopt advances in technology, and organized around the needs of service providers, not users. On the advice of Alan Enthoven (1) and others, the incoming Conservative government, under Margaret Thatcher, introduced a quasi-market in 1990 to address these shortcomings.

Quasi-market

The responsibility for purchasing health care was devolved away from government to a range of local health care organizations, including general practitioners. Large general practices and consortia of smaller practices were given budgets with which to purchase a range of community and hospital services on behalf of their patients (known as "GP fundholding"). Locally constituted "health authorities" purchased the balance of services not commissioned by GPs. At the same time, hospital and community health services were transformed into self-governing "trusts" which might compete with each other to provide the services commissioned by GPs and local health authorities.

GP fundholding was successful in increasing the range of primary care services provided to patients, reconfiguring community and hospital services to better meet the needs of primary care, and securing more rapid access to specialized hospital services for patients (2, 3). However, fundholding also gave rise to local variations in care provision that were politically unacceptable. The incoming Labour government, under Tony Blair, therefore sought to abolish fundholding while preserving its practical benefits.

Networks

The solution was to form general practices into local networks governed by Primary Care Groups (PCGs) in April 1999. PCGs had three core functions:

- to improve the health of local people and address health inequalities,
- to develop primary and community care services, and
- to commission community and hospital services (4).

PCGs were governed by a board, usually chaired by a GP and with majority GP representation. Control of the health care budgets previously managed by fundholding general practices and local health authorities was devolved step-wise to PCGs which then moved to become Primary Care Trusts (PCTs). The formation of PCTs was rapid and completed in all cases by April 2003.

PCTs have stronger public accountability mechanisms and a less prominent management role for local providers, notably GPs. The 302 PCTs in England control the bulk of the health care budget (the target is 75 percent by 2004); have responsibility for arranging the provision of all primary and community care services; commission the majority of hospital care; and lead partnerships working with local government services, including social care.

As before, GPs remain "independent" contractors to the NHS. With no direct control over GP contracts, relationships between the PCT and its general practices have mainly been based on resource sharing, mutual practical help, sharing professional knowledge and expertise, and personal contacts (5). For example, PCTs have appointed clinical governance leaders, who are usually GPs, to provide guidance and support to general practices in improving the quality of their care. Shared educational activities between practices are supported through funding that enables all practices in a locality to close for one half day a month for a joint educational session. Other activities include the development of local protocols and guidelines, promoting the use of personal learning plans and practice development plans, and the promotion of multi-practice clinical audits. Collaborative working among general practices has increased with the result that nearly all now share resources to some extent (6).

THE EXERCISE OF POWER

PCT Governance

The formation of PCTs was intended to maintain the advantages of the quasi-market (service innovation and user responsiveness brought about by GP fundholding) without its principal disadvantage (horizontal inequity in service provision). To achieve this requires striking the right balance of power between central and local governance of the health care system. Too high a degree of centralization will discourage innovation and the tailoring of services to local circumstances; too little will lead to unacceptable regional variations in the range and standard of services.

While the government is committed to the decentralization of power in principle, PCTs have little room to manoeuvre in reality. They are constrained by a host of regulatory systems that specify which services and treatments should be provided (through the National Institute of Clinical Excellence); set forth the standards to which services should be provided (through National Service Frameworks); and monitor whether these services and standards are being met in practice (through the Commission for Health Care Audit and

Inspection, CHAI). Additionally PCTs receive a mass of other policy "guidance" and "targets." Poorly performing PCTs may have their management team replaced — a threat that encourages managers to focus on centrally mandated standards and targets, rather than local health care concerns where these differ from national priorities. The PCTs that meet agreed performance standards are given greater control over budgets and services. But even then, local discretionary power is limited by the ring-fencing of budgets devolved to PCTs for national priority services.

Commentators believe that PCTs need greater autonomy if they are to fulfil their remit (7). However, as PCTs have not long been in existence, there is uncertainty as to whether they yet have the knowledge and expertise appropriately to discharge those responsibilities. This uncertainty has led to a (temporary?) paralysis in the transfer of power from government to local health care organizations.

General Practice Governance

The introduction of PCGs, and later PCTs, led to the emergence of a new stratum of GP-managers who mediate relations between rank-and-file GPs and PCT general managers (8). These GP leaders, together with the PCT managers, are the most influential voices within PCTs with non-doctors having more marginal roles (9). Whilst the leadership tends to consult rank-and-file GPs around key areas of work, the support of rank-and-file GPs is by no means universal or guaranteed (10). Outside the central managerial structure, the network periphery varies in terms of how extensively and consistently its members are involved in PCT activities (11).

PCTs must develop transparency and trust between themselves and member general practices if they are successfully to promote change (12). To these ends, PCTs have tended to use education, information-sharing, and incentives, not sanctions and disciplinary action, to deal with poor performance (13). "Clinical governance" systems have been introduced to encourage and support GPs in adopting best practice standards as articulated in evidence-based National Service Frameworks. This has moved GPs toward a more active and collegial, less permissive and individualistic, form of professional self-regulation. Tensions nonetheless arise between competing professional (GP) and managerial (PCT) interests (14). Many clinical governance leaders experience difficulty in resolving the conflict between their role in supporting and encouraging quality improvement in all practices, and their role in identifying and dealing with poor performance (13).

User Involvement

Health policy prescribes lay involvement in PCT decision making (15). Lay voices, however, have had little influence. It is not that NHS managers and clinicians are generally hostile or even indifferent to the idea of lay involvement. Rather, they have little idea what the policy means in concrete terms or how to implement it (16). They use a limited repertoire of methods. Consultations and meetings are used more than surveys, and the range of people from whom views are sought is often narrow (17). NHS information systems collect little data about users' views, and rarely use what data they do have in planning service development or setting quality standards (18). Few PCTs have been satisfactorily capturing patient and public views in the commissioning process (10). Only a minority of PCTs can identify changes in plans or policy resulting from user consultations (17). Much the same picture obtains elsewhere in the NHS, not so much because of implementation failures as because a flawed policy assumes that minority participation in committees gives users sufficient power to counter professional interests focused on the technical quality of health care, or to influence the power of managers who face incentives and imperatives unrelated to meeting users' demands (19).

IMPLEMENTING REFORM

In order to achieve change, the interests of health care professionals, notably doctors, need to be (re)aligned with those of government, and reinforced as appropriate through systems for regulating, monitoring, and remunerating medical practice.

Professional Engagement

The introduction of GP fundholding by the Conservative government in 1990 was done without GP consultation or consent, in open opposition to the British Medical Association. GPs viewed the contract as an attack on their independence and professional autonomy and believed financial restraint, rather than health improvement, was the goal (20). Fundholding was taken up quickly only by an enthusiastic minority; others joined reluctantly lest their patients be disadvantaged by the competitive edge achieved by fundholders.

The incoming Labour government of 1997 handled matters differently. They were careful to give GPs a controlling hand in the governance of the newly created PCGs — an arrangement that encouraged GP engagement with the process of abolishing fundholding and implementing new systems of governance. GP dominance was eroded by the move from PCGs to PCTs, but only after the new system had taken root — albeit a shallow root. Within PCTs, the new stratum of GP-managers governs partly by soft coercion — inviting rank-and-file GPs to engage in quality improvement and assurance initiatives but with the implicit threat of direct, less welcome, intervention should they not comply (11).

Professional Regulation and Monitoring

There has been a shift from "high" trust towards "low" trust systems of professional regulation and monitoring, signalling a greater need for public transparency and accountability in the governance of medical professionals. This shift is exemplified by the introduction of

- non-medical representation on professional governing bodies, notably the General Medical Council which licenses doctors;
- systems for detecting and remedying poor performance, coupled to enhanced powers for PCTs to suspend GPs from the local medical list;
- systems for monitoring the quality of general practice care, coupled to increased payments for high quality;
- annual appraisal and periodic re-accreditation of doctors.

The risk in moving too far towards low trust systems is that it will lead to the erosion of professionalism — the feeling of a personal responsibility that motivates doctors to work hard to meet the needs of their patients.

Financial Incentives

Payment systems need to reinforce policy objectives, creating a positive incentive for change. Conversely, if providers are financially penalized for making desired changes, then change will not occur. In accordance with national policy objectives, GP payment systems in the UK have moved from rewarding health care activity toward rewarding health care quality and outcomes.

A new national GP contract is being phased in from 2003 that will be held by the practice, not the individual GP. Thirty percent of practice income will be determined by the ability to meet quality standards across a range of 76 clinical and 56 organizational criteria, as well as 4 indicators of patients' experience of the quality of care.

Based on our current understanding of the impact of financial incentives on GP behaviour (21), these types of payment should enhance the quality of care in the targeted areas for development. As the scope of clinical care specified in the contract is very broad, many important health needs of the largest care groups will be addressed and the overall quality of primary care may rise.

Offsetting the potential gain is the risk that clinical activities that are not linked to incentives will be neglected in favour of those that are. This seems most likely in the area of acute care. A second consideration is that remunerating care for specified clinical conditions will lead to increased specialization in those aspects of care. This will provide a further impetus for role differentiation among GPs within practices and the introduction of specialized health professionals (e.g., clinical nurse specialists), thereby increasing the size and complexity of general practice teams. Continuity, coordination, and the interpersonal quality of care may diminish, particularly for patients with complex health care problems and co-morbidities. Whether these disadvantages will outweigh the advantages of improved care in targeted areas is difficult to predict.

COST OF REFORM

The UK experience has been that reform costs money, takes time and is constrained by human resource capacity and "political capital."

Capital investment is needed to fund new ways of working before old ones can be phased out and gains in efficiency realized. In order to resource NHS reforms the government has increased expenditure on health care provision from 6.7 percent of GDP in 1998/99 to 8.1 percent in 2002/3 with a further planned increase to 9.4 percent of GDP in 2007/8.

A considerable period is needed for managers and clinicians to learn how to develop and operate new organizational structures (PCTs) and systems, as well as to realign the educational and legal infrastructures required to enable reform. During periods of rapid change, the attention of frontline staff is diverted from caring for patients to instituting organizational reform (22,10). The pace and scope of reform can be such that further change becomes impossible and change itself can become a cause of diminishing performance. This is particularly a problem when change takes place against a background of shortages of doctors and nurses, as exists in the UK.

The pace of reform is further constrained by the political capital of government. A government's willingness to confront powerful vested interest groups, such as doctors, depends on how secure it believes itself to be with the electorate. The present government is facing considerable opposition from

health unions over some aspects of reform (e.g., the role of private sector finance and health care organizations in the NHS) at a time when public confidence
in the government has been called into question over its role in the Iraq war.

OUTCOMES

The way things are done has changed rapidly. In the five years since 1998,
radically new systems for managing, monitoring, and delivering primary health
care have been introduced and made operational. This is no inconsiderable
achievement.

How we think about things has also changed dramatically. GPs today are
aware that they have a personal responsibility to use resources wisely to achieve
the best possible outcomes for the whole of their patient population. There is a
greater willingness for practices to work together to improve the health of their
communities through shared knowledge, expertise, and resources. GPs are also
more sensitive to the need for greater public accountability and transparency
in primary health care provision.

Whether these reforms have actually improved the effectiveness, efficiency
or equity of health care provision in the UK is less certain. Evaluations of
discrete aspects of reform have produced encouraging findings. Quality gains
through targeted investment have been demonstrated in experimental pilots
which mimic attributes of the new GP contract to be phased in from 2003 (23).
Primary care services have been made more accessible by diversifying points
of access to include nurse-led Walk-in Centres and a national telephone advice
line, NHS Direct. Efficiency gains have been achieved through the economies
in scale and scope afforded by larger general practice teams, particularly those
in which nurses play an extended role in health promotion and chronic disease
management (24). National patient surveys show patient satisfaction with GP
services is high (25). Despite these promising indications, hard evidence of
wide-scale improvement is not yet available. In part this may be because outcomes are both difficult to measure and take a long time to materialize. More
time will be needed to judge the success or otherwise of reform.

REFERENCES

1   Enthoven AC. Reflections on the management of the National Health Service. London:
     Nuffield Provincial Hospitals Trust; 1985.
2   Goodwin N. GP fundholding. In: Le Grand J, Mays N, Mulligan J-A, editors. Learning
     from the NHS internal market: a review of the evidence. London: King's Fund; 1998.

3   Dowling B. GPs and GP fundholding in the NHS. Aldershot: Ashgate; 2001.

4   Department of Health. The new NHS: modern, dependable. London: Stationery Office; 1997.

5   Sheaff R. The development of English Primary Care Group governance. A scenario analysis. International Journal of Health Planning and Management. 1999;14:257–68.

6   Wilkin D, Dowswell T, Leese B. Primary care groups — modernising primary and community health services. British Medical Journal 2001;322:1522–1524.

7   Klein R. "The new localism": once more through the revolving door? Journal of Health Services and Research Policy 2003;8:195–196.

8   Sheaff R, Smith K, Dickson M. Is GP restratification beginning in England? Social Policy and Administration 2002;36:765–779.

9   Dowswell T, Wilkin D, Banks-Smith J. Nurses and English primary care groups: their experiences and perceived influence on policy development. Journal of Advanced Nursing 2002;37:35–42.

10   Wilkin D, Coleman A, Dowling D, Smith K. National Tracker Survey of Primary Care Groups and Trusts 2001/2002: taking responsibility. Manchester: National Primary Care Research and Development Centre; 2002. Available at http://www.npcrdc.man.ac.uk

11   Sheaff R, Rogers A, Pickard S, Marshall M, Campbell S, Roland M, Sibbald B, Halliwell S. A subtle governance: "soft" medical leadership in English primary care. Sociology of Health and Illness 2003;25:402–428.

12   Marshall M, Sheaff R, Rogers A, Campbell S, Halliwell S, Pickard S, Sibbald B, Roland M. A qualitative study of the implementation of cultural changes in primary care organisations needed to implement clinical governance. British Journal of General Practice 2002;52:641–645.

13   Campbell SM, Sheaff R, Sibbald B, Marshall M, Pickard S, Gask L et al. Implementing clinical governance in English primary care groups/trusts: reconciling quality improvement and quality assurance. Quality and Safety in Health Care 2002;11:9–14.

14   Dowling B, Glendinning C, editors. The new primary care: modern, dependable, successful? Buckingham: Open University Press; 2004.

15   Pickard S, Smith K. A "third way" for lay involvement: what evidence so far? Health Expectations 2001; 4:170–179.

16   Pickard S, Marshall M, Rogers A, Sheaff R, Sibbald B, Campbell S, et al. User involvement in clinical governance. Health Expectation 2002;5:187–198

17   Alborz A, Wilkin D, Smith K. Are primary care groups and trusts consulting local communities? Health and Social Care in the Community 2002;10:20–27.

18   Sheaff R, Pickard S, Smith K. Public service responsiveness to users' demands and needs: theory, practice and primary healthcare in England. Public Administration 2002;80:435–452.

19   Sheaff R. Responsive healthcare: marketing for a public service. Buckingham: Open University Press; 2002.

20   Calnan M, Williams S. Challenges to professional autonomy in the United Kingdom? The perceptions of general practitioners. International Journal of Health Services 1995;25:219–241.

21   Gosden T, Forland F, Kristiansen I, Sutton M, Leese B, Giuffrida A et al. Impact of payment method on behaviour of primary care physicians: a systematic review. Journal of Health Services and Research Policy 2001;6:44–55.

22   Fulop N, Protopsaltis G, Hutchings A, King A, Allen P, Normand C et al. Process and impact of mergers of NHS trusts: multicentre case study and management cost analysis. British Medical Journal 2002;325:246–252.

23   PMS National Evaluation Team. National Evaluation of First Wave NHS Personal Medical Services Pilots. March 2002. Manchester: National Primary Care Research and Development Centre; 2002. Available at http://www.npcrdc.man.ac.uk

24   Sibbald B, Shen J, McBride A. Changing the skill-mix of the health care workforce. Journal of Health Services and Research Policy 2004;9(1 Supplement):28–38.

25   Commission for Health Improvement. CHI National Patients Survey Programme: 2003 results. London: CHI; 2003. Available at http://www.chi.nhs.uk/eng/surveys/nps2003/pct.shtml

Experience Abroad II
Implementing New Zealand's Primary Health Care Strategy

Nicholas Mays and Jackie Cumming

INTRODUCTION

The implementation of the New Zealand (NZ) Primary Health Care Strategy (1), which will not be completed for at least another four to five years, is arguably the single most significant change to the scope of NZ's public system of health care since the 1940s. Government reform of primary health care, which usually involves altering the reimbursement and behaviour of general medical practitioners (GPs) in private practice, is difficult to achieve and has been attempted unsuccessfully on a number of occasions previously in NZ. GPs in NZ, as in Canada and in the UK, resisted early organizational and ownership incorporation into the public health care system, making it difficult for governments to find strategic allies in primary health care for further change. In addition, the organizationally diffuse nature of general practice has made it hard for governments to influence GPs and bring about major change in the nature and way that services are delivered.

This chapter focuses on attempting to understand the *process of implementing* the current NZ Primary Health Care Strategy rather than analyzing the merits of the strategy as a policy. The chapter is also particularly focused on the influence of the *medical profession* on this implementation process through its concern with issues of *funding and remuneration*. These foci have been chosen because the medical profession frequently exerts very significant influence over the direction, pace, and extent of health care system changes (2) and New Zealand is no exception to this pattern (3). In this case, the implementation of the strategy has major potential implications for the traditional professional and business autonomy of GPs in the New Zealand system since the state has not traditionally directly paid for primary medical care, instead subsidizing patients in their transactions with GPs. In addition, in general practice, questions of reimbursement methods have often loomed large in reforms and in the ability of governments to bring about genuine change in the nature of primary care in many countries.

The specific question posed is whether the policy adjustments made seriously risk the achievement of the government's goals. These adjustments have been made in order to implement the early stages of the strategy in response to the opposition of important interests, especially GP organizations. Most major policy change involves concessions, particularly where the support of professional interest groups is essential to the success of a policy. In the current case, the majority of GPs publicly supported the principles of the strategy, but in the early stages of implementation, significant groups of GPs expressed concerns about key aspects of the emerging funding and reimbursement arrangements. As a result, some larger organizations were reluctant to contemplate structural changes and changes in payment mechanisms. Over time, however, with concessions made by the government, and with financial incentives encouraging change, many more organizations are now becoming primary health organizations (PHOs).

Analytical Framework

The analytical framework used in the chapter is derived from Walt and Gilson's generic model of the health policy process (4). The model explains the development and implementation of health policies through the complex interplay of context, actors, and process.

- Context refers to systemic factors — political, economic, social and so on — at national and international levels. Specifically, context includes *situational factors* that are idiosyncratic or transient conditions (e.g., wars and droughts), *structural factors* that are relatively permanent features such as the type of economy or institutions, and *cultural factors* such as the assumptions and views of the population derived from the dominant religion.
- Actors is shorthand for the individuals, groups, and organizations involved in the policy process. This chapter focuses on the main GP organizations — the New Zealand Medical Association (NZMA) and the Independent Practitioner Association Council (IPAC) — which have criticized the strategy from a position of considerable influence.

• Process refers to the way policies are initiated, developed, formulated, negotiated, communicated, executed, and evaluated. The process can be represented in terms of the classical *stages* of the policy process, but, in practice, it is rarely linear (5).

The model is used to produce a preliminary account of how the content of the strategy, the context in which it was introduced, together with the actors involved and the process of implementation chosen, have shaped its implementation to date.

CONTEXT

System of Government and the Position of the Current Government

New Zealand has a unicameral, Westminster-style parliamentary system which has led to a highly centralized government system supported by a politically neutral civil service. Parliaments are elected under the mixed member proportional version of proportional representation with three-year electoral terms. The Labour Party has been the largest party in, and has dominated, two coalition governments since 1999. Since July 2002, Labour has led a government with no outright majority, but with an agreement with the Green Party for support on "confidence and supply." As a result, the Government has had to move relatively cautiously, taking left of centre supporters from other parties with it, but inherits the customary relatively top-down style of policy formation and implementation derived from before 1996 when proportional representation was introduced. To this tradition, it has added a concern to give its manifesto commitments a very high priority when developing policy once in office. Primary health care reform was a manifesto commitment of the Labour Party in 1999.

Economy and Health Spending

NZ is less wealthy than the average of the G7 countries, the world's largest economies (see Table 1). However, the economy has fared reasonably well since the mid- to late-1990s, and particularly during the last major global recession. However, long-term growth rates are lower than in Australia and many other high-income countries of the Organisation for Economic and Cultural Development (OECD). This imposes inevitable constraints on social spending, including on health services. Health spending, particularly in the public

TABLE 1

NEW ZEALAND ECONOMY, HEALTH AND HEALTH CARE

Indicator, 2001	New Zealand	Canada
GDP pc, US$ PPP*	$21,200	$29,300
Health spending pc, US$ PPP	$1,710	$2,792
Health spending as percent of GDP	8.8%	9.7%
Health spending as percent of public finance	76.4%	70.8%
Number of physicians per 1,000 population	2.2	2.1
Life expectancy at birth, years	75.7 (male)	76.7
	80.8 (female)	82.0

Note: *GDP pc = gross domestic product per capita. PPP = purchasing power parity
US$ PPP in 2001 = $30,100.

Source: OECD Health Data 2003. Available at http://www.oecd.org/

sector, has risen steadily in real terms in the 1990s as inflation has been controlled and the economy has grown at a reasonable rate (see Figure 1 and Table 1). This has given the government some possibility of expanding public health care coverage from general taxation to primary care despite the incessant demands of the public hospital sector for more resources.

Health Status

The country has a population of 3.9 million in a land mass the size of the British Isles. Eighty percent of the people live in the cities, mostly on or near the coast. The population is younger on average than that of Western European countries with 11.9 percent over 65 years of age in 2001. Almost 80 percent of the population is of European descent, mostly from Britain, with 14.5 percent indigenous Maori, 5.6 percent from other parts of the Pacific, and 3.4 percent Asians.

Average health status is very similar to that of other OECD countries such as Canada (see Table 1), though the government is concerned about the gap between Maori and non-Maori populations in life expectancy. The health of the Pacific peoples is, if anything, worse than the health of the Maori. There has been a continuous narrowing of Maori/non-Maori death rates and life expectancy since the Second World War, but recent data hint that in certain

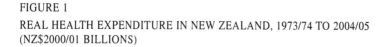

FIGURE 1

REAL HEALTH EXPENDITURE IN NEW ZEALAND, 1973/74 TO 2004/05
(NZ$2000/01 BILLIONS)

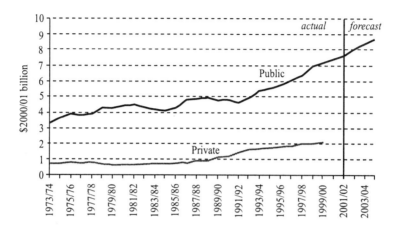

subgroups (e.g., middle-aged males), the divergence may be widening (6). Part of the rationale for focusing on primary care is to improve access to services with a view to improving overall health and closing health "gaps" between different ethnic and socioeconomic groups.

Structure and Organization of the Health Care System

The tax-financed part of the health care system was restructured in 2000 in line with Labour's manifesto pledge to remove the previous "quasi-market" (7,8). There are currently 21 District Health Boards (DHBs) responsible for planning at a local level and for purchasing and providing or arranging for the provision of the majority of health services used by geographic populations in their jurisdiction. DHBs own and manage the public hospitals, thereby verti-cally integrating the purchase and supply of acute services (see Figure 2). They also purchase a range of services from community providers. DHBs are allo-cated public tax funds according to a weighted capitation formula designed to reflect the relative needs of their populations.

At the centre, the ministry of health is responsible for policy advice to the minister of health, and for funding DHBs and monitoring their perform-ance. The ministry also purchases some public health services, maternity services, and disability support services for people aged 65 and over

FIGURE 2

STRUCTURE OF NEW ZEALAND'S PUBLIC HEALTH CARE SYSTEM, 2000-

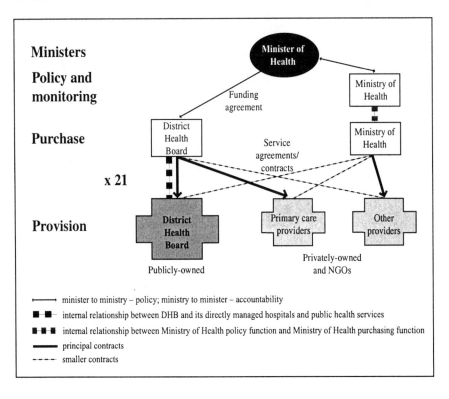

(responsibility for purchasing most of these services has recently passed to DHBs). It also oversees national screening services and some health promotion (e.g., media campaigns). The intention is that as far as possible purchase responsibilities should be devolved to DHBs subject to an assessment of their capability.

New Zealand is unique in having a separate system for meeting people's needs for health and rehabilitative services caused by injury which accounts for approximately 7 percent of total health spending and 10 percent of public spending (9). The Accident Compensation Corporation (ACC) administers a social insurance scheme that provides universal personal injury coverage. In return, people do not have the right to sue for personal injury, other than for exemplary damages. Among the services the ACC pays for are primary care services, particularly initial GP assessments and physiotherapy related to injuries. As a result, the vast majority of GPs receive public payment from ACC as well as from the general tax-financed health budget.

Most GPs work in small, privately owned group practices and act as referral gatekeepers to secondary care as in the UK and Canada. They tend, except in rural areas, not to have in-patient responsibilities.

History of Primary Care Funding

While hospital and public health services have been "fully funded" as part of a universal tax financed service since the 1940s, there has been no tradition of treating primary care in the same way. Instead, government has subsidized parts of primary care in different ways. In 1938 the NZ branch of the British Medical Association rejected full state funding of GP services and any statutory regulation of their fees. As a result, the government was forced to compromise and was only able to subsidize the private transaction of a visit to the GP and related expenditures. This drove an enduring wedge in forms of funding, organization, and careers between primary and secondary care doctors and other staff.

The initial General Medical Services (GMS) subsidy was near-universal and contributed about 85 percent of the cost of GP visits. High inflation in the 1970s and 1980s led to the erosion of the value of the subsidy which led to an increase in out-of-pocket payments. In the early 1990s the remaining public spending was refocused on people with low incomes, via the Community Service Card (CSC) and high users, via the high user health card (HUHC). Both groups continue to face an appreciable user charge of around $NZ30 (around 10 pounds sterling). In addition, there are prescription charges (first $NZ15) similar to those in the UK, but moderated for HUHC and CSC holders (see Table 2). Those without cards can pay up to $NZ55 ($C26) for GP visits, though there is no regulation of fees. Traditionally, patients faced lower co-payments for injury-related consultations under the universal ACC scheme, with the risk of cost-shifting to ACC.

Primary Health Care Benefits

In addition to the subsidies to patients set out in Table 2, there are also practice nurse subsidies to GPs which cover part of the costs to GPs of employing nurses in their practices.

GP visit fees are unregulated and vary by area depending on what local people can afford and are willing to pay, and the degree of competition between GPs. Table 2 gives an indication of the likely total costs of a GP visit against

TABLE 2

PRIMARY HEALTH CARE BENEFITS AND SUBSIDY RATES, 2001

Client Group	Subsidy NZ$		Total Client Fees NZ$	
	Per Visit	*Prescription*	*Per Visit*	*Prescription*
Over 18 years, low/middle income, family with CSC (1992)	15		35-50	
Individual high user (>12 visits in 12 months with HUHC (1992)	15		35-50	
Under 6 years (1996)	32.50	free	35-50	
6-18 years	20 if CSC 15 if no CSC		35-50	
Over 6 years, no pharmaceutical subsidy card		15		15 if drug subsidized
With pharmaceutical subsidy card		2, 0 after 20 prescriptions		2 if drug subsidized

Note: CSC = Community Service Card; HUHC = high user health card
Source: Ministry of Health/Health Benefits, Ltd.

the amount of subsidy available to particular groups of patients. If a GP pharmaceutical is not on the subsidized list or Pharmac, the government's drug buying agency, then the patient has to pay the full price.

About 40 percent of the population have a CSC, HUHC or pharmaceutical subsidy card, but it is estimated that about a quarter of those eligible do not have the necessary cards.

Current Primary Care Organization

There has never been a contractual link between GPs and the state. Thus GPs have remained small business people outside the mainstream of the public health care system. Technically the public subsidies are given to *patients* to enable them to complete a private transaction, and not to the doctors. There is no formal patient enrolment and patients are free to visit any doctor. If they are eligible for subsidized care, there is no limit on the number of visits that can be made in a specific period to a range of providers.

Currently, most primary medical care providers receive their public share of funds from the ministry via an agent (Health Benefits Ltd) which pays out general medical services patient subsidies, maternity subsidies, and pharmaceutical subsidies on an item of service basis. However, some primary care organizations are "bulk funded" (i.e., crudely capitated). These organizations typically serve low income and/or ethnic minority populations, which are informally enrolled in most cases; they came into being during the 1990s before the current primary care reforms in order to improve access in areas where conventional general practice was either weak or absent. Many of these organizations are members of a national network known as Health Care Aotearoa which strongly supports universal access to primary care services, multidisciplinary team work, and the use of capitation to allocate resources in relation to population needs.

Another development in the 1990s — the emergence of independent practitioner associations (IPAs) — contributed to the development of a more collective approach to primary care with practices collaborating, often for the first time. IPAs were spontaneous developments originated by GPs themselves to enable them better to negotiate contracts with the then regional purchasers. As a result, they are not government owned. Eighty-five percent of NZ GPs are now affiliated with IPAs, all of which manage a budget for their GP members' pharmaceutical expenditure and some for spending on laboratory investigations as well (10).

Despite these developments in the 1990s, 80 percent of GPs are still totally fee-for-service private practitioners receiving only limited public subsidy. The other 20 percent work in a range of primary care organizations or capitated practices. Some primary care organizations employ their GPs. Typically, GPs receive 40 to 45 percent of their income from public subsidies and 60 percent from patient out-of-pocket payments. This situation leads to a relatively wide distribution of GP incomes, with some practitioners doing relatively poorly compared to their peers and to those working in other professions.

As a result of these features, NZ is assessed as "intermediate" on Starfield's index of the extent of "primary care orientation" of its health care system with a score of 1.1. Using the same methods, the UK scored 1.7 at the same period in the mid-1990s (11).

CONTENT OF PRIMARY CARE REFORM POLICY

Labour's Critique of Existing Primary Care Arrangements

The Labour Party manifesto at the 1999 General Election and subsequent statements by the incoming Labour-led government amounted to a wide-ranging critique of the status quo. Labour's position and that of similarly aligned critics of the arrangements described above can be summarized in the following points:

- Care should be tax financed, free at the point of use, and made available related to need.
- Universalism in primary care will lead to better outcomes and reduced health inequalities.
- Individual targeting of public funds is inefficient, stigmatizing, cumbersome, and inequitable. The subsidy regime meant that patient charges were not related to incomes and did not cover the majority of costs. The existing patchwork of uncoordinated subsidies and fee-for-service payment inhibited teamwork.
- There was evidence of unmet need, especially in the lower socioeconomic groups, though not all research had reached this conclusion (12,13).
- Public spending on primary care was unrelated to population needs. Instead public spending was driven by the location of practitioners and patterns of patient demand. This created a diversity in patterns of provision and a large variation between and within IPAs in GMS, laboratory, and pharmaceutical spending, which could not be explained by needs (14).
- Overall, NZ spent too little of its health care budget on primary care; 59 percent was spent on hospitals while the OECD mean for hospital spending was 43 percent.
- GPs had little incentive to manage their patients' health care and their own use of secondary care, and patients, particularly the poor, had an incentive to use the hospital accident and emergency department inappropriately to avoid a user charge from their GP.

Access Problems Due to Cost

Labour's concerns, shared by many in the health care sector, were supported by the findings from population surveys. Table 3 is drawn from an international survey in 2002 of adults with health problems, but very similar results were observed in the 2001 version of this survey which looked at a random

TABLE 3

COST-RELATED FAILURE TO ACCESS HEALTH CARE, ADULTS WITH
PROBLEMS IN VARIOUS COUNTRIES

In past 2 years, did *not due to cost:*	*AUS* %	*CAN* %	*NZ* %	*UK* %	*US* %
Take up prescription	23	19	20	10	35
Get medical care	16	9	26	4	28
Get test, treatment, or follow-up	16	10	15	5	26
Get dental care	44	35	47	21	40

Source: 2002 Commonwealth Fund International Health Policy Survey of Adults with Health
Problems

sample of the *general* population in the same five countries (15). For example,
15 percent of New Zealanders in the general population had not filled a prescription due to cost in the previous year versus 7 percent of people in the UK and 13
percent in Canada (16). Twenty percent had a medical problem but had not visited
a doctor due to the cost, as against only 2 percent in the UK and 6 percent in
Canada. Among those with health problems, the percentages were higher still.

Figure 3 shows clearly how different two general tax-funded health systems — the UK and NZ — can be as regards out-of-pocket spending when one
covers and the other does not cover primary health care. The proportion of the
NZ population paying more than $1,000 in a year (11 percent) was twice as great
as in Canada (5 percent) and five times greater than in the UK (2 percent). Note
that the NZ findings are from a country where incomes are considerably lower
than in Canada, and where there is a targeting regime supposedly designed to
protect low-income and high users from the costs of health care.

NZ Primary Health Care Strategy

The Labour-led government's strategy was published in 2001 (1) after extensive consultation on a draft document with a wide range of interest groups.
The aims were:

- to emphasize the importance of population health, health promotion and
  prevention, together with developing a wider range of primary care services;

FIGURE 3

TOTAL OUT-OF-POCKET HEALTH COSTS REPORTED, BY COUNTRY, 2001

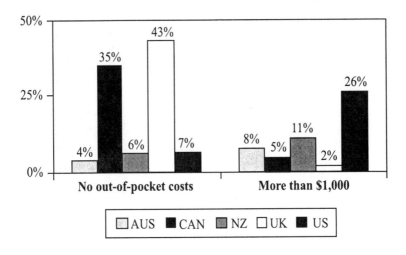

- to foster community involvement in primary care organizations;
- to involve a range of professionals and a team approach to care and decision making in primary health care;
- to improve access to first contact care for all groups in the population;
- to make primary care more affordable and provide more appropriate services;
- to improve the coordination and continuity of care;
- to fund primary care according to each population's needs.

These aims have much in common with a number of different reform efforts at the provincial level in Canada (e.g., better access for marginalized groups, wellness emphasis, multidisciplinary teams, contractual relations, shift away from fee-for-service, voluntary enrolment) (17).

In order to bring these aims about, the government proposed a shift from a number of individually targeted part-subsidies driven by demand in a private market to largely public, needs-based population funding. This was accompanied by a shift away from public payment to practitioners via fee for service to capitation similar to the approach in a number of countries. Overall, on the financing side, the government proposed a shift from predominantly out-of-pocket payment at the time of use (offset for some by use of private medical insurance) toward a predominantly prepaid system financed in the main from general taxation.

New Primary Health Organizations

New PHOs are the key mechanism through which the new primary health care system is being realized. They are required to have the following features:

- Funding is to be by needs-weighted capitation.
- They are to be non-profit, non-governmental (NGOs), with significant community governance. PHOs are to be NGOs, but with a minimum of government requirements (not-for-profit and community governance). These factors challenge the way some IPAs work; they tend to be GP owned and controlled. Government wants PHOs to behave like public bodies, but without owning them or their affiliated GP practices!
- Patient enrolment and provider affiliation is to be voluntary. The decision to allow voluntary patient enrolment via one's usual provider of primary medical care and voluntary provider affiliation means that some form of "multi-tier" system is inevitable during the transition.
- Ultimately, all patients enrolled with a PHO should be entitled to the same access to services, irrespective of their individual characteristics (e.g., income).
- Providers are to be mostly subcontracted to PHOs. Each district health board will contract with the PHOs serving its population to provide "essential" services plus additional services appropriate to the needs of the population (see Figure 4). Each PHO determines how its providers and practices are paid.

Eventually it is hoped that all patients will be enrolled with a PHO and PHOs will be funded to provide near-universal services almost all free or nearly free at the point of use. The government has not clearly defined what proportion of primary health care finance it expects eventually to provide. However, in the transition to the new system, different sorts of patients continue to attract different levels of public subsidy and, therefore, different user charges.

Patients currently remain free to choose their GP, but it has been up to the GP to decide which PHO to join. In this sense, few patients have yet to choose their PHO directly. In future, in the larger urban areas, patients may have more than one accessible PHO to choose from, though it is unclear how many PHOs will be allowed to offer their services across DHB boundaries. It is likely that ethnically focused primary health organizations will do this. A high proportion of the early PHOs are small organizations owned and run by Maori or Pacific peoples community groups. In some cases, district health boards have chosen to confine primary health organizations to covering a particular

FIGURE 4

HOW PHOs WILL FIT INTO THE NEW ZEALAND HEALTH CARE SYSTEM

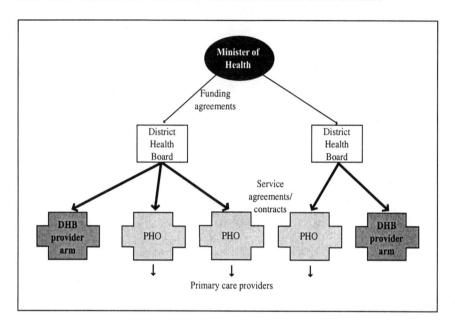

geographical location so that even if a patient switched GPs he or she might have to remain in the same PHO. In some sparsely populated areas, there are unlikely to be many PHOs regardless of the policies of the district health board.

Implications of the Content of the Strategy for Implementation

The strategy proposes a major, constitutional change (i.e., a change affecting the fundamentals, reflecting deep values, and where experimentation is diffi-cult) in the health care system. In addition, the strategy will directly affect how resources flow through primary care, creating winners and losers almost inevitably. The strategy not only seeks gradually to alter the source of finance from private to public, but also to alter the mechanism through which practi-tioners receive their public payments from fee for service at the patient level to seeking payment from capitated PHOs. Yet, this is an area where the evidence base for policy change is weak in that very little is known about the long-term impact of different reimbursement methods. On the other hand, it is known that GPs tend to prefer fee for service to capitation (18).

The strategy also represents a shift, at least in theory, from a professional contact model of primary care to more of a community model. Indeed, the fully functioning PHO has many features in common with the integrated community model of primary care identified by Larmarche et al. (19). It is interesting to note that these authors find some evidence that this model of primary care organization, similar to the Primary Care Trusts in the English National Health Service, performs better than any of the other forms that have emerged world wide. In NZ, this shift from a professionally oriented towards a community-oriented vision of primary care has been accompanied by IPA and wider GP suspicion of the community governance requirements of PHOs on the grounds that they confer power on community representatives without responsibility. Concerns about the Labour government's requirement for community governance and the not-for-profit status of PHOs relate to the fact that beneath the PHO level, practices remain as private enterprises, yet PHO board decisions are likely to be taken by people a majority of whom have no stake in the practices, but whose decisions could affect their viability. There are also criticisms that the government is trying to dictate terms to third sector organizations, although it does not own or fully pay for their activities.

All in all, this suggests that the content of the strategy is radical in the context of primary health care in New Zealand and, therefore, will be challenged in the process of implementation where it threatens cherished values and practices.

PROCESS

Policy Development

The strategy was developed through a fairly conventional process after the election of a Labour-led coalition at the end of 1999. A public consultation document outlining the main principles and elements in the new primary care system was developed by civil servants with some input from experts and a small number of individuals from the primary care sector, but with the central government leading. There followed extensive consultation on the document involving "road shows," meetings, and written responses. There appeared to be overwhelming support for the principles and goals of the strategy. The draft was then revised, agreed to by Cabinet and published by the minister as government policy. Although the strategy was claimed exclusively by the Labour-led coalition, it is worth noting that much of the thinking at official levels had already taken place under the previous National (conservative)

Government which was likely to have introduced some form of primary care reform had it remained in power.

Implementation Plan and Process

Initially, the costs of implementing the strategy and the details of how resources would eventually flow through the system and to practitioners had not been articulated, nor had the process of implementation. The published Strategy was uncosted. After estimates of the cost of implementation had been prepared, it became apparent that the new primary care system would cost an extra $850m at least, out of a total public budget of about $6.5 billion in 1998/99. Faced with such a large increase in public health spending, Cabinet determined that the strategy should be implemented in phases over eight-to-ten years at which point it seemed likely that a desirable level and share of public funding could be achieved.

Over the first three years, $410m of new money was directed to primary care, focused in the main on PHO-enrolled populations and PHO-affiliated providers so that there was an obvious incentive to take part in the new system, while allowing patients and GPs the choice of remaining outside. To build the confidence of the GPs in the new system, the new money was inflation-proofed to maintain its purchasing power, but note that the link was to prices not to wages. The previous pattern of subsidies remained, but it will not be widened or improved for those who remain outside PHOs. As a result, there should be a gradual shift away from individual targeting to funding in relation to the needs of populations of patients. It is expected that the need for low-income and high-user patients to use CSC/HUHC will decline as the amount and share of public funding rises in PHOs.

Patient co-pays remain, but are limited by local contract negotiation with the DHBs which allocate the new money to PHOs. The inflation-proofing of PHO funding is designed so that DHBs can negotiate contracts with PHOs that limit co-payment rates for defined periods into the future. Without a system of voluntary regulation of co-payments, it was not possible to obtain GP agreement to reductions. Clearly, some limits had to be put in place; otherwise the new money would simply have increased the income of GPs without reducing user charges or enabling new services to be provided. How to restrict co-payments in some way that was acceptable to practitioners, but without formal external regulation, was a major barrier to the implementation of the strategy for some time. Eventually, in 2003, an agreement was reached between the government and GP groups on the principles underlying the setting of patient fees (20).

Managing the Transition

The government's early priority over the first three years was to reduce access barriers (especially cost) for those in greatest need by allowing a minority of PHOs to qualify for higher capitations because they were serving high need populations. PHOs on the so-called Access formula receive higher capitations than those on the Interim formula to allow them to provide free or low cost access to all their patients and to increase the range of low cost services, but have to demonstrate that at least 50 percent of their enrollees are either Maori/Pacific Peoples or live in the 20 percent of the most deprived small areas in New Zealand according to the NZ Deprivation Index. These PHOs will not need to use the CSC/HUHC. It is estimated that up to 500,000 people could be covered by Access-formula PHOs out of a total population of 3.8 million. This accounts for $75m out of the $410m of new funding for primary care over the first three years of strategy implementation, 2002/03–2004/05. In addition, some practices receive Access-level funding even if the whole PHO does not qualify for the higher capitation level.

Gradually, capitations under the Interim formula will be increased as extra funds become available to bring the two formulae more into line. For example, in 2003/04, children 6 to 18 years and people over 65 years attracted sufficient funding for the PHO to give them reduced-price GP visits under both formulae. A small amount of funding was also set aside for PHOs to provide particular "Services to Increase Access."

Progress to Date

PHO formation has been faster than was generally expected. Fifty-five PHOs had been formally established by October 2003 covering an estimated 2 million enrollees out of a total population of 3.8 million. By February 2004, the Ministry of Health was reporting that 59 PHOs were operating covering about 2.5 million New Zealanders in some way (21). Individuals do not apply directly to the PHO, but enrol through their usual source of first contact care. In July 2003, 32 of the then 47 PHOs were high need and on the Access formula with eight on the Interim formula and seven out of 47 mixed, with practices on one or the other formula. Most PHOs were covering fewer than 10,000 people; seven covered more than 70,000 as the list below indicates.

- 15 <10,000 enrolled
- 13 –10 to 30,000 enrolled

- 8 – 30 to 50,000 enrolled
- 4 – 50 to 70,000 enrolled
- 7 > 70,000 enrolled

Process: Facilitating Factors

A number of enabling factors can be identified supporting the implementation to the end of 2003. It is not possible to put these in order of importance at this stage.

First, it was important, particularly at an early stage, that the primary care sector supported in principle the objectives of the strategy. Support was forthcoming before groups saw the details of the funding and transition processes. Considerable public dissatisfaction with the financial barriers to access to first contact care (the consequences of which are evident in Table 3) helped as well. For example, reducing user fees for subgroups of the population such as the under-18s or over-65s, which was announced during 2003, was popular with many, if not all, people.

Second, changes in the medical profession made the transition more acceptable. The experience of belonging to IPAs and other primary care organizations, faltering incomes for some practitioners, and the fact that younger GPs (who are increasingly female) tend to be less interested in the independent small business model of practice, have all made GPs more willing to look at being part of wider groups and to entertain the possibility of receiving more public funding. Salaried status has greater appeal than at any time in the past. Fewer new GPs are buying into practices and a sizeable proportion of members of the Royal New Zealand College of General Practitioners surveyed in 2003 reported that they intended to change their working arrangements away from self-employment in the next five years (22). In addition, from the government's perspective, the advent of IPAs, Health Care Aotearoa, and other primary care organizations before 1999 had made the sector less diffuse since the late 1980s and the negotiations easier.

Increased public funding for primary care has attracted many GPs since some have seen their incomes falling in recent years and, therefore, are more interested in a change of funding base, despite reservations about the sustainability of government funding sources. Many primary care organizations serving low income, rural, and Maori communities were set up in 1990s with bulk-funding arrangements inadequate for the demands they faced. These organizations, such as the Health Care Aotearoa network, have seen the strategy and new funding as a way of accessing a fairer, more realistic level of funding in relation to their populations' needs. The NZ economy has done relatively well through the recent global recession and extra public money has been available for the health sector. The existence of, and the political presence, of these organizations has provided the government with models for, and strong supporters of, change.

Third, several aspects of the government's approach won over some potential critics. From the outset the government was committed not to regulate user charges by statute, but to find a more informal way to restrict their rate of increase; there was never a threat to nationalize (i.e., own) general practices; and the government was flexible about certain aspects of the requirements for PHOs (e.g., population size). Thus PHOs are envisaged as exclusively NGOs (unlike English NHS Primary Care Trusts which are statutory authorities) (23). As another concession, the government agreed to bring forward by a year the funds to reduce co-pays for all those over 65 years to July 2004, in order to reduce the odds of GPs on the Interim formula losing patients to GPs on the better funded Access formula. In addition, the government found additional resources to increase the management fee for small and moderate-sized PHOs and put a cap on the number of out-of-PHO visits for which any PHO/provider could be financially liable.

Finally, a degree of bi-partisan support has assisted the implementation process. The National Party has criticized the detail of the strategy, but has said little against the overall aim of improving access to a more capable primary care sector. In part, this is because the party is uncertain about policy after a second successive election defeat and preparatory thinking on reforming funding and access to primary care was undertaken by civil servants on their watch before the 1999 election, though no decisions had been taken on reform.

Re-introduction of Individual Targeting: The "Care Plus" Concept

If willingness on the part of the government to respond to criticism of the plans, for example, by a faster introduction of money to reduce user fees for the over 65s, has helped smooth implementation so far, the "Care Plus" pilot has been the major concession designed to keep influential GP groups supportive of the strategy.

The piloting of the Care Plus concept proposed by the IPA Council (IPAC) (24) represents a way of bridging the new and the old systems of allocation during the transition period. It is intended to allay the concerns of some GPs about sensitivity of capitation at a small population level. An individual enrolled will attract an enhanced capitation payment if he or she

- has had more than six GP/ED visits in the previous year or more than two unplanned hospital admissions,

- requires terminal care,
- has two or more chronic conditions,
- is on "active review,"
- or has a HUHC.

Up to 5 percent of any PHO's population can be designated as Care Plus patients. Care Plus payments go directly to the practices where patients are registered and are earmarked to be spent on individual patients.

The Care Plus pilot shows the government willing to compromise in response to concerns and to implement a potentially feasible alternative form of resource allocation. From the perspective of *improving* access for hard-to-reach groups, the major problem with the concept is that it links resources to patients already known to have health requirements for time and support, but does nothing for PHOs with large numbers of patients with previously unmet needs. It also relies heavily on GP discretion in identifying suitable patients. Furthermore, it risks hindering the eventual implementation of the government's desired end-point of needs-weighted capitation funding of PHOs. Arguably a combination of the HUHC and the advent of free care for the over-65s from 2004 would deal with most of the cases that concern GPs. However, in small PHOs, with large numbers of patients with chronic conditions, or at practice level, the concept introduces the first element of what may become a blended payment approach. Blended payment for primary care is regarded by many as preferable to simple capitation (12).

Process: Obstacles to Implementation

The process has encountered many obstacles and objections to date. Predictably, most GPs and GP representatives have either objected to or been suspicious of any hint of reduced autonomy, particularly to set user fees. The tradition of fee for service, subsidized private practice is not to be swept aside easily or quickly without huge sums of extra public funding not currently available. DHB caps on fee levels have been seen as an arbitrary limitation on GPs' incomes, especially where these have been falling recently. Some GPs mistrust Labour's motives vis-à-vis the small business, for-profit model of NZ general practice on the grounds that the government will be unwilling to pay properly for an alternative state-controlled and financed model.

Another obstacle has been fears among GPs about the potential impact of the lengthy transitional period on the viability of their practices, for example, through competition for patients. Patients may prefer to enrol with practices on the Access formula while these practices receive higher funding and can afford to levy lower fees. GPs practising in or near the catchments of high-need PHOs feel particularly vulnerable. GPs in general are unwilling to see themselves become dependent on government for their livelihood in case government funding withers and/or demand increases far in excess of the extra funding. There are also criticisms from practices which fear that they will lose from capitation.

Perhaps the most widely heard criticism, and potentially a substantial obstacle which the government has had to work to remove, has been of "inequities" in the transitional funding arrangements with "high need" people in "low need" areas failing to find an Access PHO and vice versa. There are also concerns about the variations in fees charged in this lightly regulated environment. GPs are not alone in their concern lest the transitional distinction between the funding of different PHOs becomes an enduring part of the system, for example, because there is not sufficient public funding to reach a near-universal system.

Behind many of these detailed process objections, are fundamental conflicts between different principles of fairness — most notably, between selectivity with individual targeting and universality with population-based allocation on the basis of areas' relative needs — and different views about their impact. Some GP and patient groups have been slow to grasp and accept the policy of funding according to the relative needs of PHOs' populations rather than in relation to workload and/or costs of care generated by individuals.

Lessons for Primary Care Reform Implementation

What may we learn from this preliminary case study of a strategy under implementation? First, it is clear that simultaneous change to the source of finance (private to public) method of reimbursement (FFS to capitation), governance (professional contact to community-controlled model), and scope of services in a sector is intrinsically risky and likely to generate opposition, particularly when the state does not fully pay for the services in question. Second, while such radical changes need to be phased accordingly, this can be hard to sustain over a long transition. Third, in-principle support at the outset can be misleading, when key stakeholders lack detailed information on methods of funding and on likely winners and losers! Fourth, compromises and a degree of flexibility are almost certain to be needed to support the implementation process, so it may be wise to anticipate the "pinch points" and have (limited) compromises or alternative development paths worked out in advance. Finally, the continuing influence in a new setting of established, taken-for-granted ways of working should not be underestimated. In this case, the assumptions derived from the past policy of subsidizing identifiable individuals rather than funding organizations to provide services to populations, have proved tenacious and may yet survive a reform process designed specifically to remove such individually targeted public support.

REFERENCES

1   Minister of Health. The New Zealand primary health care strategy. Wellington: Ministry of Health; 2001. Available at http://www.moh.govt.nz/

2   Tuohy CH. Accidental logics: the dynamics of change in the health care arena in the United States, Britain and Canada. New York and Oxford: Oxford University Press; 1999.

3   Fougere G. Struggling for control: the state and the medical profession in New Zealand. In: Hafferty FW, McKinlay JB, editors. The changing medical profession: an international perspective. New York and Oxford: Oxford University Press, 1993. p 115–123.

4   Walt G, Gilson L. Reforming the health sector in developing countries: the central role of policy analysis. Health Policy and Planning 1994; 9:353–370.

5   Hill M. The policy process in the modern state. Third edition. Harlow: Prentice Hall; 1997.

6   Brown MC. Policy-induced changes in Maori mortality patterns in the New Zealand economic reform period. Health Economics 1999; 8:127–136.

7   *New Zealand Public Health and Disability Act,* 2000.

8   Cumming J, Mays N. Reform and counter-reform: how sustainable is New Zealand's latest health system restructuring? Journal of Health Services Research and Policy, 2002; 7(suppl 1):46–55.

9   Ministry of Health. Health expenditure trends in New Zealand 1990-2001. Wellington: Ministry of Health. Available at http://www.moh.govt.nz/

10   Malcolm L, Wright L, Barnett P. The development of primary care organisations in New Zealand: report to the Treasury and Ministry of Health. Wellington: Ministry of Health; 1999.

11   Grant CC, Forest CB, Starfield B. Primary care and health reform in New Zealand. New Zealand Medical Journal 1997;110:35–39.

12   Malcolm L. Inequities in access to and utilisation of primary medical care services for Maori and low income New Zealanders. New Zealand Medical Journal 1996;109:356–358.

13   Peacock D, Devlin N, McGee R. The horizontal equity of health care in New Zealand. Australian and New Zealand Journal of Public Health 1999;23:126–130.

14   Malcolm L. An evaluation of pharmaceutical management and budget holding in Independent Practice Associations and General Practices. A confidential report prepared for the Transitional Health Authority and Pharmac. Lyttelton; Aotearoa Health; 1997.

15   Blendon RJ, Schoen C, DesRoches C, Osborn R, Zapert K. Common concerns amid diverse systems: sicker adults' views and health care experiences in five nations. Health Affairs 2003;22:106–121.

16   Schoen C, Doty MM. Inequities in access to medical care in five countries: findings from the 2001 Commonwealth Fund International Health Policy Survey. Health Policy. In press.

17   Hutchison B, Abelson J, Lavis J. Primary care in Canada: so much innovation, so little change. Health Affairs 2001;20:116–131.

18   Hurley J, Hutchison B, Giacomini M, et al. Policy considerations in implementing capitation for integrated health systems. Policy Synthesis. Ottawa: Canadian Health Services Research Foundation, no date. Available at http://www.chsrf.ca/funding_opportunities/commissioned_research/polisyn/pdf/pses-impcap_e.pdf

19   Lamarche PA, Beaulieu M-D, Pineault R, Contandriopoulos A-P, Denis J-L, Haggerty J. Choices for change: the path for restructuring primary healthcare services in Canada. Final report. Ottawa: Canadian Health Services Research Foundation; 2003. Available at http://www.chsrf.ca/search_e.php

20   Minister of Health. Agreement reached on Primary Health Organisation detail. News release. 14 May 2003. Available at http://www.beehive.govt.nz/viewDocument.cfm?DocumentID=16768

21   Ministry of Health. Primarily. February 2004; 8. Available at http://www.moh.govt.nz/publications/newsletters/primarily

22   Austin C, Glensor P. Barriers to access. Presentation to International Forum on Common Access to Health Care. Wellington; 29 January 2004.

23   Minister of Health. Minimum requirements for primary health organisations. Wellington: Ministry of Health; November 2001.

24   IPAC. Options for introducing new primary health care funding. Wellington: Independent Practitioner Association Council; 2002. Available at http://www.ipac.org.nz/public/news/NewsAndPubsItemViewPrint.aspx?id=38

Health Care Reform Strategies in Cross-National Context

Implications for Primary Care in Ontario

Carolyn Hughes Tuohy

INTRODUCTION

As we seek to understand the opportunities for and constraints upon primary care reform in Ontario, there are lessons to be learned from the broader experience with health care reform agendas in other jurisdictions in the 1990s and early 2000s. While the health policy agenda in the 1990s had many common elements across Organisation for Economic and Cultural Development (OECD) nations, the strategies adopted varied widely in the scope and the pace of change attempted. Roughly, these strategies fall into three categories. "Big-bang" strategies attempted to establish, in one step, a comprehensive framework for change. "Blueprint" strategies attempted to set out a comprehensive framework to be accomplished over time through a series of steps. And "incremental" strategies made adjustments to the existing system without an overarching framework. The choice of strategy and the likelihood of its enactment depended upon factors in the broad political environment, but the success of the implementation of that strategy, depended on factors in the health care arena itself, and in particular on the structure of interests. This paper will draw upon the examples of Australia, Canada, the Netherlands, New Zealand, the United Kingdom and the United States to illustrate the dynamics at work (1).

NATIONAL STRATEGIES OF HEALTH CARE POLICY REFORM

In the last decade of the twentieth century, the policy debate in the health care arena in most advanced nations swirled around the questions of the extent to which and the ways in which the health care system needed to be "reformed." Driven by fiscal pressures, the rate of increase in public spending on health care slowed on average across OECD nations through much of the 1990s. Potentially more significant than this fiscal restraint, moreover, was the development of a set of agendas for redesigning health care programs and institutions. While these reform agendas varied, they had in common a concern with the structure of incentives embedded in programs of health care delivery and finance, and the declared objective of redesigning programs to provide incentives to efficiency and effectiveness. Pursuing this agenda meant moving beyond the blunt instruments of budget constraint and cost-shifting that governments had relied on in the past, and attempting to include micro-level considerations of the relationships between providers and purchasers of care.

Table 1 summarizes the types of strategies adopted in each of the nations reviewed in this paper, and the results. Interestingly, neither a big-bang, nor a blueprint, nor an incremental approach seems in itself to have been more successful in achieving its intended result. Of the nations that attempted big-bang reform, one (Britain) succeeded in implementing a somewhat tempered version of the changes originally proposed; one (New Zealand) enacted sweeping change from which it successively retreated; and one (the United States) failed to enact reform proposals at all. The jurisdictions that took a blueprint approach (the Netherlands and some US states) found themselves stalled after having achieved change in some subsectors of the health care arena or for some income categories of the population. And those nations that attempted incremental change (Australia and Canada) had mixed success in different subsectors. In fact, regardless of the strategy chosen, change appears to have been most effective where governments succeeded in engaging a subset of actors in the health care arena in the process of implementing health care reform — albeit in ways that had not been specifically anticipated at the outset.

TABLE 1

STRATEGIES OF HEALTH CARE POLICY REFORM

Strategy Type	National Example	Result
Big Bang	United Kingdom	Tempered adoption of internal market Subsector change (fund-holding)
	New Zealand	Rollback of internal market Subsector change (budget-holding)
	United States (federal)	Failure to enact universal coverage through "managed competition"
Blueprint	Netherlands	Stalling of "managed competition" Subsector change (social insurance reform)
	United States (some states)	Stalling of universal coverage Subsector change (Medicaid expansion)
Incremental	Australia	Subsector change (private insurance subsidies)
	Canada	Subsector change (hospital restructuring)

Understanding Health Care Reform: The Choice of Strategy

Whether or not a nation attempted bold policy change in the 1990s, let alone experienced the likelihood of success, bore little relationship to overall trends in spending on health care, or to the share borne by the public treasury (2). Rather, the strategic approach to health care reform in a particular nation depends on factors in the broader political environment. Given the entrenchment of interests in the health care arena and the high public salience of health care, making such changes carries great political risk. Hence governments are likely to approach health care reform with varying degrees of caution, depending on their political circumstances.

- Big-bang approaches require the combination of two factors: the government of the day must believe that it can muster its *authority* on a scale that will allow it to succeed; and health care reform must be sufficiently central to its political agenda that it has the political *will* to incur the risk of undertaking it.

- Blueprint reforms are likely to attempted where a government has the *will* to make large changes, but cannot mobilize *authority* necessary for a big bang approach.
- Incrementalism is essentially a default option in which the political will to make large changes is lacking; for example, because doing so would be inconsistent with a broader agenda or because the risks of doing so are deemed too high.

Table 2 summarizes the political conditions at the time reform strategies were adopted in each of the nations under review.

TABLE 2
CONDITIONS FOR ENACTING REFORM

Strategy Type	National Example	Political Conditions
Big Bang	United Kingdom	Unitary parliamentary government structure Majority government in third successive mandate
	New Zealand	Unitary parliamentary government structure Majority government
	United States (national level)	Federal: bicameral congressional government structure at national level Presidency and both Houses of Congress controlled by same party by narrow margins
Blueprint	Netherlands	Unitary parliamentary government structure Coalition government
	United States (state level)	Federal: bicameral congressional government structure at state level Divided government in some states; same-party control of both houses of legislature and state house in others
Incremental	Australia	Federal parliamentary government structure — relatively strong central government Majority governments at national and state levels
	Canada	Federal parliamentary government structure — poor climate of federal-provincial relations Majority governments at national and provincial levels

The Big-Bang Approach: Britain, New Zealand and the United States

The decision by a government to attempt big-bang reform is an uncommon event. The two factors that lead to such a decision — the government's belief in its capacity to mobilize *authority,* and its political *will* to make major change in the health care arena — rarely coincide.

Nonetheless, at least one of these conditions for a big-bang approach — the ability of the government of the day to muster authority on a broad scale — is more likely to occur in some systems than in others. It is most likely in systems that provide relatively few "veto points" for opponents, and therefore in systems with features such as a unitary (non-federal) structure, a parliamentary model that concentrates authority in the executive, an electoral system that favours the emergence of a majority party, and a tradition of party discipline that minimizes intra-party dissent. Even in such systems, the mere ability of government to mobilize authority is not a sufficient condition for it to proceed with big-bang change. It must also form the *will* to take the political risks involved — because systems that concentrate authority also concentrate accountability, and it is difficult for governments in such systems to diffuse the blame for unpopular reforms (3).

It is not surprising that in two of the three nations under review here in which big-bang change was attempted — Britain and New Zealand — all of these conditions were present. In both of these unitary Westminster systems, a governing party with a strong ideological bent formed the political will to take on health care. In Britain, it was a Conservative government in its third successive majority mandate that adopted a set of "internal market" reforms aimed at organizing the system around "purchaser" and "provider" entities and requiring them to contract with each other. In New Zealand, "internal market" reforms were also adopted by a conservative (National Party) majority government, after a period of experimentation with market-oriented reforms in sectors other than health care under a predecessor Labour government (4).

It is more rare but not impossible for big-bang change to occur even in systems that lack the consolidation of authority that characterizes parliamentary systems in unitary states. In the United States, with a federal structure, a congressional system that divides authority between the legislature and the executive, and a tradition of very weak party discipline, big-bang change has occurred on a number of occasions. Most notably, in the health care arena, it occurred in the 1960s when the Democratic landslide in the 1964 federal elections gave that party the presidency with a super-majority in the popular vote, as well as super-majorities in both houses of Congress; and governmental health insurance in the form of Medicare for the elderly and Medicaid for welfare recipients was introduced. It is also possible for sweeping change to occur through the mobilization of bipartisan support in the US system, as occurred with the passage of tax reform legislation in 1986.

President Bill Clinton clearly had the political will to introduce universal health insurance through "managed competition" as a central component of his "New Democrat" agenda, and made a commitment to health care reform central to his presidential campaign. He chose an approach to reform that built upon the existing employer-based model, mandating employers to provide health insurance for their workers, and requiring state governments to establish regional health alliances to contract with private insurers to offer insurance to those without employer-based insurance. His party, moreover, not only controlled the White House but also had a majority in both Houses of Congress. But Clinton's ability to mobilize the necessary authority was highly tenuous. He entered office with only a 43 percent plurality of the popular vote and with a Democratic majority in the Senate less than the 60 percent necessary to prevent effective Republican vetoes through procedural manoeuvering. In this relatively weak position as president, he could succeed in a major initiative such as health care reform only through bipartisan compromise or through creating a "bandwagon" momentum that would draw supporters to a winning cause. Strategic judgments made by the Clinton administration, however, militated against either of these outcomes (5). In the end, Thomas Jefferson was right — in the American system "great innovations should not be forced on slender majorities" — and the Clinton health care reform proposal went down to defeat (6).

The Blueprint Approach: The Netherlands and US States

Blueprint approaches are typically adopted where no one set of political actors (such as a majority government) can mobilize sufficient authority to take a big-bang approach, yet comprehensive reform is still the goal. In such circumstances, agreement on a blueprint, incorporating elements desired by different parties and interests, may be negotiated, to be implemented on a phased basis. This was the approach adopted in the Netherlands in the context of coalition governments in the late 1980s and 1990s, and by several American states in the early 1990s in attempts to achieve bipartisan compromise.

In the Netherlands, the intent was to replace the existing system, in which health insurance coverage was structured by region and by income category and was divided between "sickness funds" and private insurers, with an overarching framework of "managed competition" integrating all insurers.

These proposals bear the mark of a coalition government. The end — universal scope — appeals to the left; while the means — regulated competition — appeals to the right. (Indeed, just such an attempt at left-right appeal, though not the process of negotiated compromise nor the phased approach, underlay the Clinton reforms in the US.) The reforms were proposed by a commission established by a centre-right coalition government in 1987 and essentially endorsed by the centre-left coalition government (with a social-democratic health minister) that assumed office in 1991 (7).

Phased blueprint approaches to health care reform were also adopted by some American states in the early 1990s, including Minnesota, Oregon, and Washington. Again, this blueprint strategy appeared to make sense in the political circumstances of the time, which required the building of liberal-conservative coalitions both across and within political parties (1).

Incrementalism: Australia and Canada

In both Australia and Canada, changes in the public policy framework for health care financing and/or delivery followed a more incremental pattern. The conditions for a big-bang or a blueprint approach were simply not present. Both of these nations are federal states in which responsibility for health care is shared between national and sub-national governments. Hence the process of mobilizing the authority necessary to make comprehensive reforms is more complicated than in unitary states. There are, however, important differences between the two federal systems. While provincial governments in Canada have far greater fiscal leverage in the health care arena than does the federal government, Australian state governments are largely dependent on the Commonwealth (the federal government) for health funding (8). Canadian provincial governments operate hospital and medical insurance plans under criteria established in federal legislation as conditions for federal financial transfers; in Australia the medical insurance plan is operated by the Commonwealth government, while state governments own and operate public hospitals with Commonwealth funding.

In Australia, then, the federal government has a stronger role in health care than is the case in Canada and is more able to take unilateral action. In the 1990s, however, for the first time in decades a change in government at the Commonwealth level did not lead to a comprehensive change in health policy: the Liberal-National Party Coalition government elected in 1996 (and re-elected in 1998) did not dismantle the policies of its Labour predecessors, but sought to strengthen private elements of the system on an incremental basis — largely through increasing public subsidies for private insurance (9).

In the 1990s, policy change in Canada could be characterized as "incrementalism under fiscal duress" (10). This was a period of intense focus on deficit reduction, and accordingly of cuts to program spending, at both federal and provincial levels. In health care, real per capita public spending began to decline in 1992, troughed in 1996 and 1997, and then began a sharp trajectory of increase. If public spending had instead followed a pattern of steady secular increase from 1992 to the point it reached in 2000, about $30 billion more (current dollars) would have been spent collectively by federal and provincial governments over the period (11). The mechanisms of fiscal constraint were blunt, and left the essential design of the system unchanged. There was no experimentation with "internal market" reforms as in Britain and New Zealand, and no deliberate shifts in policy to favour private finance as in Australia. No government was willing to bear the political risks of "going it alone" to tamper with Canada's most popular social program, without the political cover provided by a federal-provincial agreement. And in the highly strained climate of federal-provincial relations in the 1980s and 1990s, no such agreement was possible.

At the federal level, transfer payments were reduced in a series of federal budgets beginning in 1985. At the provincial level, governments also confined themselves primarily to blunt budget instruments to slow the growth of the health care budget and to reallocate within it. They did intervene to restructure the hospital system; and in all provinces except Ontario (a large exception, representing about 40 percent of the Canadian health care system) they established or increased the authority of governmentally appointed or elected regional boards for the governance of hospitals and other institutions. These boards continued to function at arm's length from the provincial government, however; and members were more likely to see their roles as that of community representatives rather than agents of the provincial government (12).

In summary, the basic parameters of both the Canadian and Australian systems remained largely intact in the 1990s, while incremental changes were made. Choices about the nature of those changes, and the course of their implementation, were very much shaped by the design of the existing systems in ways that will be discussed in the next section.

IMPLEMENTING HEALTH CARE REFORM: STRATEGIC ALLIANCES

Regardless of whether governments adopted a big-bang, blueprint or incremental approach to health care reform, their success was contingent on their ability to find allies within the health care arena itself. And the nature of those alliances shaped the course of implementation.

The possibilities for such alliances depend upon the structure of interests in the health care arena — a structure that in turn depends on the design of the prevailing policy framework. In particular, it depends on the way in which the boundary between public and private finance is drawn, and the resulting balance of influence across the state, private finance, and key health care providers. Essentially four models for drawing this boundary can be identified:

1   Parallel public and private systems: For a given range of services, often only a small subset of services in profitable "niche" areas, a separate privately financed system exists as an alternative to the public sector. The primary axis of accommodation in the arena is between health care providers and the state, with private insurers playing a relatively marginal role.

2   Co-payment: Across a broad range of services, financing is partially subsidized through public payment, with the remainder financed through out-of-pocket payments and/or private insurance. In such systems, providers deal with a mix of sources of finance for any given patient, the basis for accommodations between providers and payers is more fragmented, and private insurers may play a significant role.

3   Group-based: Certain population groups are eligible for public coverage; others rely on private insurance. In such systems, providers move from one type of payer to another as they move from patient to patient. This also fragments the basis for accommodation between providers and payers, although it may provide the basis for separate accommodations around particular patient populations. Private insurers are major players.

4   Sectoral: Certain health care sectors are entirely publicly financed; others privately financed. In such systems, there is a strong base for accommodation between the state and those providers whose services are publicly funded, while fragmenting the base for broader accommodations. Private insurers are confined to certain sectors, typically not involving "core" services.

The nations under review here exemplify these models to greater or lesser degrees (Table 3). Their experience with implementing health care reform reflects those differences.

The Implementation of Big-Bang Reform: Britain and New Zealand

Prior to their attempts at big-bang reform in the 1990s, the British and New Zealand systems showed some important similarities and differences — and the differences were to prove crucial to the dynamics of change in the 1990s.

TABLE 3

CONDITIONS AFFECTING THE IMPLEMENTATION OF REFORM

Strategy Type	National Example	Public-Private Boundary	Structure of Interests
Big Bang	United Kingdom	Parallel public and (niche) private systems	State/provider accommodation
	New Zealand	Hybrid: Parallel public and (niche) private systems plus widespread co-payment	Divided: state/providers/ private insurers/individual payers
	United States (federal)	Group-based plus widespread co-payment	"Hyper-pluralism" plus state/provider accommo- dation around Medicare
Blueprint	Netherlands	Group-based	"Social middle ground": social insurance funds, physician associations, private insurers
	United States (states)		"Hyper-pluralism" plus state/provider accommo- dation around Medicaid
Incremental	Australia	Hybrid: Parallel public and (niche) publicly subsidized private systems plus widespread co-payment	Divided: state/providers/ private insurers/individual payers
	Canada	Sectoral: medical and hospital exclusively publicly financed; other sectors mixed or exclusively private	State/provider accommoda- tion re medical and hospital services

In both Britain and New Zealand, hospitals were publicly owned and managed as well as publicly financed, offering universal access to hospital services on a first-dollar-coverage basis, although private hospitals offering a limited range of services existed in a parallel private system. Specialist physicians practised in public hospitals on a salaried basis, but most also supplemented their in- come through fee-for-service private practice. Private insurance was available for patients opting to be served in the private sector. Beyond these fundamental similarities, however, the most important differences concerned the organization and financing of general practitioner services. In Britain, general practitioners, while formally maintaining the status of "independent contractors," were funded on a capitation basis through local bodies, and patients faced no user charges for GP services. In New Zealand, GPs practised on a fee-for-service basis. Public payment for general practitioner services was conceived from the inception of the system in 1938 as a means-tested subsidy to patients, and always left upper-income patients responsible for a significant proportion of the fee. Over time, the level and extent of public subsidy failed to keep pace with the growth of medical fees, until by the 1980s public funding accounted for only about half of total expenditure on primary care.

A second difference between the two systems concerned the governance of the hospital system. The nationalization of hospitals and their reorganization within a structure of regional hierarchy constituted a key feature of the establishment of the British National Health Services (NHS) — one that was highly contested at the time but which endured through several reorganizations of the NHS in subsequent decades. In New Zealand, in contrast, existing local structures of hospital governance were left in place when the system was nationalized in the late 1930s.

These differences in financing and organizational design had important implications for the political dynamics of each system. The comprehensiveness of the British system bound health care providers into a close accommodation with the state, defined by what Rudolf Klein has termed an "implicit bargain," in which the profession accepted the state's authority to determine the overall budgetary parameters of the system while the profession retained autonomy to make resource allocations through the exercise of clinical judgment within those parameters. The system was webbed with clinical and managerial networks that, while complex, reached levels of maturity that reduced transaction costs for decision makers — an important feature in a budget-limited system. In New Zealand, in contrast, the accommodation between providers and the state was much less embracing. The relationship between local structures of hospital governance and central decision makers was a tense one, marked by periodic failed attempts by the centre to reorganize the hospital system (13). Even more significant was the fact that general practitioners, who accounted for well over half of New Zealand's practising physicians, became more and more dependent over time on private sources of finance, whether from patients out-of-pocket or from private insurers.

In these two national contexts, the attempts at "internal market" reform played out quite differently. In Britain, a broad policy blueprint outlining dramatic change was moderated in its implementation as it was absorbed by established networks.

In New Zealand, the process of policy change itself was highly volatile, as a number of policy shifts and reversals followed in rapid succession.

In Britain, the reforms formally split the established NHS hierarchy into "purchasers" (reconstituted Health Authorities) and "providers" (independently constituted hospital and community trusts), and required them to enter into contractual arrangements. But the component pieces re-established their networks even as their negotiations became more explicit. And general practitioners moved to a more central position with the surprising popularity of what was initially seen as a rather minor aspect of the reforms — the option for GPs to become "fundholders," with capitated budgets with which to buy drugs and approximately 20 percent of hospital and community services for their enrolled patient populations (14). By 1997, there were 3,500 fundholding practices acting as purchasers for approximately 50 percent of the population for a limited range of health care services (15).

GP fundholders, indeed, became allies of the government in cementing the irreversibility of the internal market reforms. When Labour assumed power in 1997, it maintained the essential features of the purchaser/provider split while changing the language in which it was described. "Contracting" became "commissioning" and "competition" became "collaboration." Moreover, Labour universalized the concept of GP fundholding under another name with the establishment of Primary Care Commissioning Groups, the precursors to Primary Care Trusts (PCTs), as the key purchasers in the system. Primary Care Trusts are essentially consortia of general practices and community nurses, with authority and budgets to enter into long-term "service agreements" with providers of hospital and community care. The role assigned to nurses in this structure is notable, and builds upon a tradition of nursing involvement in the governance of the British National Health Service. The PCTs effectively absorbed the fundholder model, and are taking over the purchasing role of the health authorities (16).

In contrast to the British case in which the internal market reforms were absorbed and tempered by established networks, in New Zealand a more tenuous accommodation between health care providers and the state was further strained by dramatic attempts at reform. The institution of the purchaser/provider split was seen as yet another episode in the ongoing contest over the organization of hospital governance. The purchasing bodies, moreover, were created from scratch, and not through the restructuring of established entities as in Britain. This meant that there were no established networks to mediate the implementation of the reforms. Even more important, the GPs who had increasingly fallen outside the scope of the provider-state accommodation could not easily be recruited to support the reforms.

The New Zealand reforms, instituted in 1993, required government-appointed purchasers (initially four Regional Health Authorities and subsequently one central Health Funding Authority with four branches) to bargain and enter into contracts with competing public and private health service providers. The management structure of public hospitals was reorganized on a Crown-corporation model. New Zealand also adopted its own version of GP fundholding, known as "budget-holding." In the New Zealand version, physician groups of varying size were given capitated budgets by the relevant health authority to cover the cost of specified services for their patients such as drugs, diagnostic texts, x-rays, etc. — but not hospital services in the British mold. Unlike GP fundholders, moreover, New Zealand budget-holders continued to function on a fee-for-service and effectively private basis for the bulk of their practice.

The result was a very rocky implementation process marked by a series of policy reversals. Some aspects of the reforms — the institution of user charges in public hospitals and a proposal for managed competition between regional health authorities and private purchasers were quickly abandoned. Under the coalition government elected in 1996, the process of dismantling the reforms accelerated. With the election of a minority Labour government in 1999, the process of dismantling the internal market reforms proceeded to completion, and the system returned essentially to its pre-1993 configuration comprising the Ministry of Health and locally elected District Health Boards, centred around their respective public hospitals.

Despite this general rolling back of the internal market reforms, there may prove to be one "sleeper" effect with some British echoes. General practitioner "budget-holding" gained popularity over time. Substantial numbers of general practitioners voluntarily opted to be budget-holders for laboratory services and pharmaceuticals, and many joined together in "independent practice associations" (IPAs). By the end of 1996, 60 percent of general practitioners were budget-holders in IPAs (17). While not as comprehensive as the British fundholding model, the spread of budget-holding did slowly begin to provide a base for primary care reform. The primary health care reform project launched under the Labour government in the early 2000s is leading to an extension of the budget-holding model to establish Primary Health Organizations (PHOs). The reform proposals, greeted with cautious support from the medical profession (18), envision a system whereby patients enroll with a given practice, and practices would receive a capitation-based subsidy for each enrolled patient.

Reform in the Wake of Big-Bang Failure: The United States

In the wake of the failure of the Clinton proposals in 1994, health care reform reverted to "politics as usual." That is, it revolved around changes to already established programs, and particularly around the Medicare program for the elderly and disabled (which accounts for about 40 percent of total public spending on health care). Since the early 1980s, the politics of Medicare, with its huge fiscal implications, had been intimately bound up with congressional budgetary politics. In the 1990s, these budgetary politics were played out on a terrain of intense partisan hostility and what Allen Schick has termed a "hyperpluralism" of interests resulting from turbulent change in the American mixed market for health care (19).

In this context, the budgetary politics of Medicare has revolved around three themes: attempts to reduce payments to providers as the common denominator of a bipartisan consensus; partisan contests over the opening up of the single-payer Medicare program to include private insurers; and myriad proposals for extending Medicare to include coverage for out-of-hospital pharmaceuticals, culminating in the adoption in December 2003 of a complex optional entitlement. The fragmented political economy of American health care seems likely to continue to generate politically induced insurance labyrinths and market turbulence.

The Stalling of a Blueprint: The Netherlands and American States

In the Netherlands, the elaborate blueprint of reform adopted in the early 1990s stalled in its early stages. As van de Ven and Schut point out, the reforms were adopted as a compromise package at the outset (7). But what was not appreciated at the time was that, in a succession of coalition governments, progress would be very difficult unless *each step along the way* were as balanced as was the full package — an almost impossible design problem. The grand scheme of universal health insurance through managed competition was abandoned in 1994, when a complex coalition led by Labour, but including the rightist Liberals and excluding, for the first time in 20 years, the centre-right Christian Democrats, assumed office.

Nonetheless, significant progress has been made in certain sub-arenas – notably social insurance and prescription drugs. Again, these reforms were shaped by the structure of interests in the Netherlands. In the Dutch group-based system, providers move from the world of social insurance to the world of private insurance as they move from patient to patient. But these two worlds are quite well-defined within an overarching regulatory framework. Accommodations occur within a "social middle ground" populated by relatively large and cohesive bodies: the sickness funds, the physician associations, private insurers, etc., in which organizations serve both private interests and public purposes (20, p 68–69).

The most significant change in the 1990s was the abolition of regional monopolies for sickness funds, which were freed to compete with each other for subscribers and to contract with physicians across the country. The major effect of these reforms was a reshaping of the "social middle ground" in health care. A number of sickness funds merged; a number of hospital mergers occurred; some sickness funds acquired hospitals; and regional cooperation among providers was reinforced and extended (20, 21). It is negotiation among these emerging horizontal and vertical alliances that is now driving developments in Dutch health care.

Similar problems were experienced in the US states that adopted blueprint approaches. In each case, these plans were stalled or rolled back as a result of partisan change in government and the fraying of political support over time. The 1994 elections shifted the centre of political gravity to the right at both state as well as federal levels. The Republicans gained both houses of legislature in Oregon, and one house in Washington state; and the Democratic majority was reduced in Minnesota. Consequently, the first-phase reforms were scaled back in Oregon and Minnesota, and later-stage reforms were repealed in all three states (22). In Oregon, an ambitious plan to extend public coverage to a broader range of low-income beneficiaries by rationing the scope of services covered was implemented — but further steps toward insuring the working poor through employer mandates were forestalled.

In the wake of these failures to proceed with their blueprints, states reverted to classically incremental approaches to change, expanding or contracting their Medicaid programs at the margin as the fiscal climate improved or worsened (23). While there are substantial disparities across states, the result of this resiliency has been an expansion of coverage: between 1991 and 2001 the number of low-income Americans covered by Medicaid increased from 27 million to 47 million (24). State governments could contract with managed care organizations to provide Medicaid coverage for enrollees, who essentially had no option. By 2002 more than 58 percent of Medicaid enrolment was in managed care arrangements, as compared with 14 percent of Medicare beneficiaries (25), and managed care organizations had become key actors in the Medicaid program.

Implementing Incremental Change: Australia and Canada

In Australia and Canada, political circumstances generated neither a big-bang nor a blueprint approach to health care reform, but rather led to a series of incremental changes. The nature of the changes needs to be understood in the context of the structure of interests in the health care arena, and particularly in terms of the relationship between the medical profession and the state.

Canada's sectoral distinction between public and private means that the health care providers traditionally at the core of the system — physicians and hospitals — are bound into an exclusive relationship with the state in a system of effective bilateral monopoly. In the foundational bargain between the profession and the state, prices for medical services are centrally negotiated and publicly paid. In return for giving up individual discretion over price, physicians secured a generous level of remuneration — not in comparison with the United States, but in comparison with the other countries treated here (26). They maintained a system with a relatively high level of clinical autonomy, relatively low transaction costs, and pivotal influence in the system through structures of effective co-management at both hospital and central levels.

In Australia, the terms of the profession-state bargain have been quite different since governments have deliberately sought to maintain a tripartite system of finance involving public finance, out-of-pocket private payment, and private insurance across a broad range of services. Individual physicians maintain discretion over price, as well as considerable clinical autonomy. They are not wholly dependent on the state for remuneration: they can bill patients at rates of their own choosing above the insured benefit. In return, however, they have accepted a considerably lower level of public remuneration than is the case in Canada. Even when private sources are added, this means that medical incomes have been well below those in Canada. Transaction costs are also higher, although physicians have increasingly accepted the trade-off of avoiding these costs through "bulk billing" (that is, billing the Medicare plan directly, and agreeing to accept the Medicare rebate as payment in full) (27). The Australian bargain thus fractured the base for an accommodation between the profession and the state. And by leaving open the private finance option, it obviated the need for a key quid pro quo such as exists in the Canadian bilateral monopoly — namely, a central place for the medical profession in policy-making bodies.

Incremental policy changes in Canada and Australia reflect these different structures of interests. In Canada, the approach was to constrain payments to providers even while increasingly involving them in joint policy-making bodies. In Australia, reforms were focused primarily on increasing the role of private insurance. Australia's attempts to blend public and private financing of medical and hospital services had resulted in an unstable system marked by economic uncertainty for private payers, be they individual patients or insurance funds. There had been a steady decline in the percentage of the population who took up private insurance, from 80 percent in 1970 to 50 percent in 1984 to 30 percent in December 1998 (28). In the late 1990s, in an attempt to staunch the flow away from private insurance and to preserve a blended tripartite structure of finance, the Coalition Commonwealth government instituted a series of measures involving the public subsidization of private insurance. While these policy changes appear to have stemmed the exodus from private insurance and may even have reversed the trend (29), it is questionable whether the very large public subsidy (estimated in 2000 at A\$2.19 billion per year, equivalent to about 6 percent of total public spending on health care) is an effective use of public funds. Duckett and Jackson have shown, for example, that directing an equivalent expenditure toward public treatment in public hospitals could fund a shift of about 47 to 65 percent of private hospital patients into the public sector (30).

In Canada, incremental change meant attempting to elaborate the accommodation with medical and hospital providers even while constraining their budgets. Canada's distinctive way of defining the boundary between public and private finance exacerbated the effects of this fiscal constraint. It meant that the brunt of the reductions in public spending was borne by those elements — medical and hospital services — that had traditionally been publicly perceived to be at the core of the system. Fiscal constraint, indeed, amplified the effects of the "passive privatization" of health care that was already occurring as technological changes shifted services out of hospital, to a world in which private finance played a much larger role. And it placed the central accommodation between health care providers and the state under unprecedented pressure.

In the hospital sector, government found some allies among those institutions who stood to gain through restructuring. With the exception of the restructuring of hospital facilities, governments relied on the blunt exercise of their monopsony power through budget-capping. Hospital budgets were still essentially based on historical experience and across-the-board changes (albeit with some attempt to develop formulae rewarding efficiency in performance) and not on negotiated packages of service (31). Furthermore, the hospital-physician relationship, based on independently constituted medical staffs, remained unchanged.

Medical practice remained outside the scope of restructuring exercises; and independent private fee-for-service medical practice remained the cornerstone of the system. Bargaining relationships remained essentially between provincial governments and provincial medical associations. Following the past pattern of blunt budgetary controls, which left the fine levers of decision making to physicians, governments sought to negotiate (and where they could not negotiate they imposed) global caps on their physician services budgets. The agenda of those bargaining relationships, however, expanded in the 1990s as provincial governments sought to elaborate their accommodations with the medical profession. By the mid-1990s, bipartite joint management committees with equal representation from government (including in most cases a representative of the finance ministry) and the medical association had been established in seven provinces. (A functionally equivalent arrangement had existed in Quebec since the early 1980s.) Such joint management arrangements formalized and arguably increased the influence of the medical profession; but they also involved the medical associations in controversial decisions that led to fissural tendencies within their memberships (32). Despite periodic flirtations with support for private-sector options, however, medical associations at both the federal and provincial levels remained formally committed to the principles of the *Canada Health Act,* and have in general focussed their arguments on the need to increase public investment in the health care system.

CONCLUSIONS AND IMPLICATIONS FOR PRIMARY CARE REFORM IN ONTARIO

This paper might be read as chronicling the triumph of incrementalism in public policy. It does not. Big-bang strategies (as the UK experience attests) and blueprint strategies (such as the experience of the Netherlands attests) have a greater impact in reshaping health care systems than attempts to make incremental changes might have done. Arguably, by establishing a grand vision, each of these strategies challenged actors in the health care system to respond. While the British big-bang vision was tempered in implementation and the Dutch blueprint has (so far) stopped short of its intended outcome, the purchaser-provider split and the role of GPs in purchasing across a broad spectrum of health care services in Britain, and the horizontal and vertical alliances among sickness funds and health care providers in the Netherlands constitute substantial changes that would not have occurred in the absence of an overarching framework.

But for both big-bang and blueprint strategies, some caveats must be issued. The conditions for big-bang approaches are rare, and are more likely (though not exclusively) to be found in institutional systems with relatively few veto points such as unitary states and Westminster parliamentary systems. They are vulnerable to strategic misjudgments leading to loss of momentum and failure, as the case of the Clinton reform in the US demonstrates. And although big-bang strategies may establish new terms for negotiating with established interests, those negotiations will determine how the changes are implemented, as the contrasting experiences of Britain and New Zealand with "internal market" reforms demonstrate. The British reorganized existing structures and long-established networks reknit themselves. In New Zealand, some key structures were created from scratch, and never found a footing.

A phased-in blueprint appears more promising in a context in which a number of competing parties and interests need to be accommodated, as was the case in the Netherlands and in some American states. Even here, however, there are a number of cautions. A coalition of support for the reforms must be maintained at each step along the way. This is both a political and a policy design problem. Political circumstances may change (as was the case in the American states, and to a lesser extent in the Netherlands). It is also very difficult to design policy steps in such a way that each can command support on its own, rather than as part of an overall package enacted at once. This was the experience of the Netherlands, which found itself stalled once reforms had been enacted in the social insurance sub-arena, before being extended to the sub-arena of private insurance.

Incrementalism appears, in a sector as dense with established interests and political, economic and institutional resources as health care, to be the "normal" or "default" strategy: it occurs when neither the mobilization of authority necessary for a big-bang approach nor coalition-building around a blue-print strategy is possible. But as is the case for the other approaches, strategic alliances are central in bringing about change. Indeed, what is remarkable about each of the three broad strategies of health care reform is the extent to which successful implementation depends on *strategic alliances within subsectors*, regardless of the comprehensiveness and speed of the approach attempted. What varied in the cases reviewed in this paper, and significantly so, was the leverage that those subsector alliances had on the system as a whole.

This observation raises an important proposition. Government programs of coverage for health care are delivered through complex webs of expert providers and, in some cases, financial intermediaries. The capacity of state actors to bring about change is limited by their reliance upon these other actors in order to mount public programs. State actors can, however, choose to ally with different groups within the web of interests by using different policy instruments. GP fundholders in Britain (and to a lesser extent GP budget-holders in New Zealand), physician and hospital Medicare providers and Medicaid managed care providers in the US at federal and state levels respectively, social insurance funds in the Netherlands, private insurers in Australia, and medical and (select) hospital providers in Canada all played the role of strategic allies shaping the implementation of health care reform.

What can this review of cross-national experiences imply for the strategic approaches to primary care reform in Ontario? Is this a moment for big-bang reform? Would a phased blueprint be the wiser approach? Or should the incrementalism of past decades be continued?

Let us first consider the prospects for big-bang reform. In the 1980s and 1990s, as argued above, the conditions for big-bang reform were simply not present in Canada. Mobilizing the necessary authority would effectively have required federal-provincial agreement, an almost impossible task in a broad climate of federal-provincial relations dominated by wrangling over jurisdictional issues. Given the popularity of medicare, moreover, the political risk of making major changes in the health care system was too high for any one government to form the political will to act unilaterally.

The events of the 1990s fundamentally changed each of these conditions. The sharp decline in real per capita public spending represented a substantial fiscal saving at a time when governments at all levels were struggling to balance their books. But that fiscal swing proved devastating to public confidence. Polls taken in 1988, 1998, and 2001 show that the proportion of Canadians who believed that "only minor changes" were needed to the system declined dramatically from about 56 percent in 1988 to about 20 percent in 1998 and did not recover with the increases in public expenditure in the late 1990s and early 2000s (33).

These developments also meant that fiscal quarrels over health care came to define the agenda of federal-provincial relations, rather than being held hostage to broader constitutional disputes. And the shaking of public confidence meant that inaction vis-à-vis the health care system came to be politically riskier than action. Arguably, indeed, a window of opportunity for major change in health care policy did open in the early 2000s with the confluence of these factors. In the deliberations and reports of governmentally commissioned inquiries in Saskatchewan, Quebec, and Alberta, and of the federally appointed Romanow commission and the federal senate inquiry under Senator Michael Kirby, a broader range of options for change were considered (including in some cases a greater role for private purchasing) than had been the case since the establishment of medicare in the 1950s and 1960s. In this historic moment of opportunity for big-bang change, governments chose to *reconfirm* the basic parameters of the Canadian single-payer model, while recognizing the need to address three key areas of priority — primary care, home care, and coverage for catastrophic drug costs. Through federal-provincial "framework agreements" in 2000 and 2003, the federal government agreed to increase its base transfers to the provinces for health care, and also established targeted funding arrangements in each of these three areas (34).

Of these three areas, primary care may well be the most promising, both because of its leverage on the system as a whole and because of the potential to form crucially important strategic alliances in support of the *implementation* of reform. Experimentation with various models for the delivery of primary care (differing in the range of services comprehended and in the degree to which they are based in community clinics or professional practices) is proceeding in all provinces to a greater or lesser degree (35). And in a number of provinces, including Ontario, there are footholds of support within medical organizations for the building of strategic alliances. There is by no means unanimity within the medical profession on this (or any other) issue, but there is sufficient support to suggest that a voluntary approach structured with appropriate incentives can gain widespread acceptance — as in the case of GP fundholding leading to Primary Care Groups in Britain and, it appears, GP budget-holding leading to Primary Health Organizations in New Zealand (36).

There remains the question as to the strategy that is best able to build upon these footholds of support. Following a phased-in blueprint approach appears promising, given the desire to arrive at a common framework while accommodating competing parties and interests. But as experience in the Netherlands and the American states has shown, it is very difficult to design a blueprint that can maintain the coalition of support at each step along the way, particularly as political circumstances change. Would it be wiser then to revert to the default position of making incremental change as opportunities arise?

Some very sensible advice in this regard comes from Brian Hutchison, Julia Abelson and John Lavis. They argue for a strategy that comprises "two complementary approaches in parallel." One involves the "unbundling" of the components of primary care reform into "those elements with broad stakeholder support (for example, enhanced clinical information systems)" that could be implemented first on a system-wide basis while efforts are made to build consensus on other elements. But lest progress on such a blueprint stall in the early stages, Hutchison and his colleagues also suggest an incremental approach that "embrace(s) ... pluralism of organizational and funding models. Opportunities to move forward could be offered to those ready to embrace innovation, without attempting to impose change on the remainder." Key to the success of these parallel strategies will be the effectiveness of demonstration effects and, as Hutchison and colleagues note "thoughtful and rigorous evaluation" (37).

This combination of approaches has several promising features. In its "blueprint" aspects, it has the potential to maintain a degree of momentum toward future steps lacking in a purely incremental approach. But it is also realistic enough not to hold all progress hostage to consensus on a blueprint, and to allow for opportunistic incrementalism even if that means a plurality of models.

Challenges clearly remain. Can sufficient momentum in fact be maintained through such a combination of approaches? Hutchison and his colleagues
themselves acknowledge the danger that the implementation process could
become "bogged down" in the complexity of different organizational arrangements. Furthermore, focusing on strategic alliances with family physicians
leaves incorporation of non-medical providers, especially nurses, as a key un-
resolved issue. Continual alertness to these challenges should shape the strategy.
The alternative to proceeding in this way, however, may be failure to realize
the opportunities for reform that present themselves within the distinctive Canadian context.

REFERENCES

1   These comparisons are more fully elaborated in Tuohy CH. "Big bangs, blueprints and
     incrementalism: a cross-national perspective on patterns of policy change in health care,"
     a paper prepared for the Conference on New Challenges for Welfare State Research,
     Sponsored by Research Committee 19 of the International Sociological Association,
     Toronto, Ontario, August 21-24, 2003.

2   The average annual increase in total per capita health spending from 1980–1992 was
     about 9.3 percent in the US, 8.6 percent in Canada, 8.0 percent in Britain and 5.7 percent
     in New Zealand. Schieber G, Poullier J-P and Greenwald LM. Health system perform-
     ance in OECD countries, 1980-1992. Health Affairs 1994;13(4):102.

3   Pierson PD and Weaver RK. Political institutions and loss imposition: the case of pen-
     sions. In: Weaver RK and Rockman BA, editors. Do institutions matter? Washington:
     Brookings Institution, 1993. p 110–150.

4   Brown M. New Zealand health care financing "reforms" perceived in ideological con-
     text. Health Care Analysis 1996; 4:293–308; Gauld RDC. Big bang and the policy pre-
     scription: health care meets the market in New Zealand. Journal of Health Politics, Policy
     and Law 2000;25(5):815–844.

5   Tuohy CH. Accidental logics: the dynamics of change in the health care arena in the
     United States, Britain and Canada. New York: Oxford University Press; 1999.

6   Quoted in Heclo H. The Clinton health plan: historical perspective. Health Affairs
     1995;14(1):86–95.

7   van de Ven PMM and Schut FT. The Dutch experience with internal markets. In: Jérome-
     Fôrget M, White J and Wiener JM, editors. Health care reform through internal markets.
     Montreal: Institute for Research on Public Policy; 1995:95–118.

8   The Commonwealth government provided about two-thirds of total public health ex-
     penditure in Australia in 1995/96. See Podger A and Hagan P. Reforming the Australian
     health care system: the role of government. Canberra: Commonwealth Department of
     Health and Aged Care; 1999. p 12.

9   Gray G. Maintaining medicare: rhetoric or reality. New Doctor 2000. 1999/2000; 72-
     (Summer).

10   Naylor CD. Health care in Canada: incrementalism under fiscal duress. Health Affairs
     1999;18(3):9–26.

11   Tuohy CH. The cost of constraint and the prospects for health care reform in Canada. Health Affairs 2003;21(3):32–46.

12   Lomas J, Veenstra G and Woods J. Devolving authority for health in Canada's provinces: III. motivations, approaches and attitudes of board members. Working Paper 96-4. Hamilton, ON: McMaster University Centre for Health Economics and Policy Analysis; 1996.

13   Laugesen M. Institutionalized localism: the politics of hospital reform in New Zealand, 1935-1995. PhD thesis, University of Melbourne, Australia, 2000.

14   See the report of the Audit Commission, What the doctor ordered: a study of GP fundholders in England and Wales. London: HMSO; 1996 p 6. Standard fundholders did not purchase the following sorts of hospital care: emergency admissions, inpatient mental health, costs above £6,000 per annum for any patient, accident and emergency, maternity, and medical inpatients.

15   Department of Health. The new NHS. London: HMSO; 1997. figure 1.

16   LeGrand J. Further tales from the British National Health Service. Health Affairs 2002;21(3):116–128.

17   Malcolm L. GP budget holding in New Zealand: lessons for Britain and elsewhere? British Medical Journal 1997;314(7098);1890–1893.

18   New Zealand Medical Association. Health strategy document welcome, but more details needed. Press Release. June 1, 2000.

19   Schick A. How a bill did not become law. In: Mann TE and Ornstein NJ, editors. Intensive care: how congress shapes health policy. Washington DC: AEI/Brookings; 1995. p 227–272.

20   van der Grinten TED. Conditions for health care reform: changing the policy system of Dutch health care. In: Proceedings of the 4-country conference on health care reform and health care policy. Ottawa: Health Canada; 1996. p 68–69.

21   van Doorslaer E, Schut FT. Belgium and the Netherlands revisited. Journal of Health, Politics and Law 2000;25(5):878.

22   Experience in other states was similar. In Kentucky, for example, plans to extend state coverage to all those below the federal poverty line were not implemented. It must be noted, however, that one state that adopted a version of a big-bang approach — Tennessee, which attempted to extend state-subsidized coverage to all uninsured residents — encountered severe implementation difficulties and closed enrolment in the program. For a fuller discussion of state-level reform, see Tuohy (5) p 85–86 and works cited there.

23   Boyd DJ. The bursting state fiscal bubble and state medicaid budgets. Health Affairs 2002;22(1):46–61.

24   Rowland D and Tallon JR. Medicaid: lessons from a decade. Health Affairs 2002;22(1):138–144.

25   Hurley RE and Somers SA. Medicaid and managed care: a lasting relationship? Health Affairs 2002;22(1):77; Brown LD and Sparer MS. Poor program's progress: the unanticipated politics of Medicaid policy. Health Affairs 2002;22(1):40.

26   Average physician income at PPP in 1990 was $89,923 in Canada — almost 60 percent higher than the average for Australia, the UK and New Zealand, but only about 55 percent of the average in the US. OECD database 1999.

27   The proportion of services that were "bulk billed" rose from 49 percent in 1985/86 to 72 percent in 1997/78. Deeble J. Medicare: where have we been? Where are we going?" The Gordon Oration. Canberra: National Centre for Epidemiology and Population Health, Australian National University; 1999. p 4.

28   Hall J. Incremental change in the Australian health system. Health Affairs 1999; 18(3):99.

29   The percentage of the population with private health insurance increased from 30.1 percent in December 1998 to 31.2 percent in December 1999 to 45.8 percent by September 2000. Private Health Insurance Administration Council. Available at http://www.phiac.gov.au/

30   Duckett SJ and Jackson TJ. The new health insurance rebate: an inefficient way of assisting public hospitals. Medical Journal of Australia 2000;172 (May 1):441.

31   Some provincial governments contracted with hospitals to provide specified volumes of a few given procedures, such as coronary artery bypass surgery. The contracting mechanism was most popular among regional health authorities in Alberta.

32   Katz SJ, Charles C, Lomas J, Welch HG. Physician relations in Canada: shooting inward as the circle closes. Journal of Health Politics, Policy and Law 1997;22(6):1413–1432.

33   Blendon RJ, Schoen C, DesRoches CM, Osborn R, Scoles KL and Zapert K. Trends: inequities in health care: a five-country survey. Health Affairs 2002;21(3):182–191.

34   Federal/Provincial/Territorial First Ministers 2003. First Ministers' Accord on Health Renewal. Available at http://www.scics.gc.ca/pdf/800039004_e.pdf

35   Canadian Institute for Health Information. Health care in Canada 2003. Ottawa: CIHI; 2003. p 19–26.

36   Mays N, Cumming J. Experiences abroad II: implementing New Zealand's primary health care strategy. In: Wilson R, Shortt SED, Dorland J. editors. Implementing primary care reform: barriers and facilitators. Montreal and Kingston: School of Policy Studies, Queen's University and McGill-Queen's University Press; 2004. p 49–71.

37   Hutchison B, Abelson J, Lavis J. Primary care in Canada: so much innovation, so little change. Health Affairs 2001;20(3):127.

From Cinderella to Belle of the Ball

The Politics of Primary Care Reform in Canada

Antonia Maioni

If health care — and politics — were simple, there would be little debate about the value of primary health care. Indeed, recent cross-national data analysis supports the conclusion that strong primary care systems are associated with improved population health (1). But, just as the promotion of basic educational skills has become difficult in the fast-paced environment of research-driven reform and the informatics revolution, so too must basic primary care principles compete with other models of medical care and organization. This is true in Canada as elsewhere, where three decades of primary care rhetoric have not, until relatively recently, led to much in the way of reform outputs.

How is it, then, that we are witnessing a primary care renaissance in Canada, as policy-makers, providers, and patients focus on the promotion of primary care as a front-burner agenda item for health care reform? How did primary care, which for so long languished in relative obscurity, become a focal point of reform aspirations across provincial health care systems?

This paper draws together themes in the larger literature on the politics of health to illuminate policy change in the case of primary care. The first section reviews the evolution of primary care in the context of the Canadian experience in health reform. The next sections explore the role of interest groups, and of political institutions, in explaining change in health care. The chapter then looks at the implementation of primary care reform and the transformation of this Cinderella into the belle of the health reform ball.

THE LONG AND WINDING ROAD TO PRIMARY CARE REFORM

The international community tends to date the emergence of a primary care "vision" with the 1978 joint WHO/UNICEF Declaration of Alma-Ata, that affirmed access to basic services as a "fundamental human right" and defined primary health care as a policy goal for both developed and developing countries (2). The policy community in Canada had a profound impact on this vision, mainly from the principles enunciated in the 1974 Lalonde report that emphasized environments and health care organization as the building blocks of better health outcomes; the emphasis on the social determinants of health in the Ottawa Charter of 1986 again underscored the linkage between population health and primary care (3).

Primary care has a very broad definition, which makes it complicated to analyze, but most definitions involve an emphasis on integrated approaches to health that include prevention as well as care, community resources and access points, and integrated teams of care providers. In the Canadian experience, primary care reform ranges from the community based to the physician led, and has been associated with both structural reform — devolving care out of institutional settings — but also payment reform in which the system of fee-for-service payment to physicians is also under review (4).

Prior to the introduction of public hospital and medical insurance, rudimentary primary care was often the only type of care to which many Canadians, in particular those that lived in rural areas, had access. In other cases, those without insurance would only access health care services for acute illnesses. Despite the nostalgic portrait of services dispensed by family doctors and community nurses, the integration of such care was not widespread in Canada.

Part of the impetus toward the public health care model in Canada was the belief that health care delivery could be better organized — not just insured — through a coordinated and publicly administered system. The political bargains struck to realize the public model, however, entrenched the political barriers to change in primary health care. The initial split between hospital and medical insurance and the implementation of public hospital insurance first seems reasonable given that hospital bills were of concern to individuals, and that hospital funding could be more easily "socialized" than doctors' fees. This was clearly the gamble that Tommy Douglas's Co-operative Commonwealth Federation (CCF) government was ready to embark upon in the 1940s. When medical services became publicly insured in the 1960s, several constituencies in the social-democratic movement (including labour) pushed for capitation or salaried physicians (5). But this was rejected in favour of a key concession: the "core bargain" — in political terms — struck between physicians and the state was to allow physicians to retain small group, fee-for-service practice (6). This "private practice, public payment" arrangement (7) was at the heart of the medical insurance model that encouraged the physician-centred delivery of health care, including primary care. This was reinforced by the *Canada Health Act*, which defined "comprehensiveness" in terms of medically necessary care, delivered by hospitals and health care professionals.

Primary care thus became part of larger backdrop to public payment and private provision of services, making it difficult to develop integrated models of health care delivery. And, in due course, primary care reform was overtaken by cost control mechanisms and then explicitly linked to these efforts. In their review of primary care in Canada, Hutchison, Abelson and Lavis (8) identify three "waves" in this process: the development of alternative models in organization and funding in the 1970s; the expansion of the scope of providers beginning in the mid-1980s; and the pilot projects launched in most provinces since the mid-1990s. Much of this development parallelled regionalization, to some degree, in the health sector, leading to the devolution of responsibility for funding and organization of health services.

More recently, provincial health care commissions and two "national" commissions — the Commission on the Future of Health Care in Canada led by Roy Romanow, and the Standing Senate Committee on Social Affairs, Science and Technology chaired by Michael Kirby — have moved almost in tandem in their focus on primary care reform. The principal critique in these reports was that primary care services were dominated by a sickness rather than wellness model, and that integration and continuity of care were essential to reforming the entire health care system (9). Innovations in primary care are now underway in pilot projects in Alberta, Ontario, British Columbia, Saskatchewan, and Quebec.

The Quebec Experience in Primary Care

The Quebec experience is instructive in understanding some of the roadblocks to primary care reform, and puts the current unblocking of such reform into perspective. Primary care started earlier and got farther, faster in Quebec than in other provinces, and yet, primary care reform long remained the Achilles heel of the health care system in the province.

The movement toward primary care began in 1966, the same year that Parliament passed the *Medical Care Insurance Act*. That year, the Castonguay-Nepveu Commission was established, with the specific mandate to review and recommend policies on health and social services in Quebec, including medical insurance, service provider organization and remuneration, and a plan for the regionalization of services. In 1970 and 1971, the commission's report became the basis for the *Loi sur la santé et les services sociaux*, guided by the principles of primary care and the integration of health and social services based on community-centred access to such services (10). It was also a reform that was based on the regionalization of services in an explicit attempt to decentralize decision making (11).

This type of "visionary" reform was fueled by an ideological discourse of social democracy, but the political reality of implementation did not correspond to these ideals (12). Physicians retained their special status as non-salaried professionals in the health sector and remained wary of the network of community health and social service clinics where general practitioners worked on a salaried basis in tandem with provider teams. The CLSC (Centres locaux de services communautaires) network put into place in the early 1970s was infused with a primary care vision that promoted integrated care. Although the CLSC network now covers the entire territorial and population reach in Quebec, these clinics have not become integrated providers of health care services in all settings (especially in urban areas) nor the front door to primary care for a majority of the population. The disconnect between the community and integration models of primary care reform and professional autonomy was palpable, as doctors initially boycotted the CLSCs and set up alternative general practice clinics. The Rochon Commission report in 1988 and subsequent reform proposals for a "virage ambulatoire" (ambulatory care) in 1990 again emphasized regionalization and integration, but the hurdles to primary care reform remained intact (13).

As the mid-1990s ushered in a period of severe fiscal crunch for health care establishments, the focus on primary care as a quality concern was subsumed under the immediate needs for cost control; the levers that were used in Quebec (including hospital closures) did not, in this respect, differ from those used in other provinces. The release of the Clair Commission report on health care in 2001 once again heralded CLSCs as a central component of the reorganization of front-line services based on the creation of new networks of family physician practices using capitation on the basis of enrolments. The first pilot projects for these Family Medicine Groups (Groupes de médecine familiale) were soon underway, in which the FMG negotiates with the local CLSC for the delivery of front-line services. Although there is concern from physician associations, the objective is to have at least 80 percent of family practitioners join these groups. In effect, although the initial investment in the new network is considerable, the FMGs are now being promoted as a way of addressing shortages of family physicians in Quebec, rather than as a way of integrating care.

Since the Quebec CLSC model differs from primary care models in other provinces because of the explicit emphasis on community-based care, the family practice reforms will also differ from the kinds of primary care alternatives envisioned in the other provinces, which until now have been physician-led or professional models. Yet, the Quebec experience shows that there are several challenges to primary care reform, and that implementation can be fraught with roadblocks.

POLITICS AND THE POLICY PROCESS: WHY POLITICAL "WILL" DEPENDS ON A "WAY"

What are the conditions that could lead to political change in primary care reform? The above overview raised some pivotal barriers and critical junctures. Much of the literature on social policy development is differentiated between the "old" politics of the welfare state in its "golden age" of program expansion and spending (14) and the "new" politics based on retrenchment in an era of "permanent austerity" (15). In the former era, health care reform in most settings, even the US, was motivated by opening access to care — in both organizational and financial terms — as widely as politically feasible. In the current era, health care reform has been overlaid by cost concerns in which the impact of primary care reform takes on a different meaning and import. In the United States, for example, integration of care through health maintenance organizations is motivated by cost concerns; while in the United Kingdom, the implementation of Primary Care Trusts is facing delay due to the considerable start-up costs associated with such reform (16).

Whose Voices Are Heard? The Role of Interest Groups, Social Movements and Political Parties

Interest groups and social movements can act as catalysts for, or opponents to, change. A basic question however is, where does demand or resistance to change come from? Most public health issues are caught in a public goods conundrum (17): the benefits may be diffused to a large but unorganized group, but a smaller but more tightly organized group (or special interest) may be more powerful in blocking or shaping the policy outcomes. The larger group can be championed by an interest group: the case of organized labour as a counterweight in health care is a good example. Labour movements in both Canada and the US lobbied long and hard for public health insurance despite the "free rider" effect; that is to say, that the benefits of such reform would accrue to a larger population than their members alone. Today, in Canada, unionized health care workers are caught in the same dilemma as other special interests in the health field: how to effectively protect their interests while contributing to the overall coherence of the health care system. Although organized labour and the constituencies it represents, for example, Canadian nurses' associations, champion primary care reform, this has not had the same mobilizing impetus as in the past.

This diffuse benefit/specific costs dynamic can sometimes be punctuated by the mobilization of diverse constituencies or social movements that coalesce around a perceived threat to general or specific public health issues, such as the anti-tobacco coalition (18). Such movements are difficult to mobilize, however, as shown in the experience of single-payer heath insurance in the US. Political change requires persistent and sustained demand but also a window of opportunity that can propel issues through the policy process (19). Public support for primary care reform remains ambiguous mainly because it is now perceived as part of the quest for cost control and efficiency, rather than as an essential reform for the maintenance of the public system. Seen in this light, individual preferences will reflect the perceived effects on personal concerns about access to care and wariness to change, and may trump more collectively oriented attitudes toward the health care system as a whole (20).

Faced with this diffuse demand, concerted opposition to change can be effective, especially when such opposition is led by those who supply the goods in question. An important challenge in primary care reform, indeed in health reform in general, has been the conciliation of health care providers, in particular physicians, into the design and redesign of health care systems. Historically, interest groups that represented physicians' lobbies were opposed to state intervention in the medical field, and this holds true across most health care systems and polities (21).

Physician resistance is a factor in the health care story in Canada; some of it before the fact (pre-emptive) and some of it after political decisions have been reached (the two "doctor's strikes" associated with twentieth century health care reform in Canada were both launched after the passage of legislation). In the case of primary health care, it has been argued, the "contractual relationship" between public payers and physicians is the "critical barrier" to primary care reform (22). And organized labour in health care settings is also a factor since the structural change involved in primary care reform will also be borne by health care workers. These disruptions, even if temporary, further underline the fact that adjustment costs are a prime motivation for resisting change. In Canada, however, hospitals and the workers within them have been easier targets for bold reforms, such as hospital insurance in the 1950s and the forced restructuring of the 1990s.

Political parties also play a crucial role as transmission belts for ideas and interests between society and the state. Partisan politics matters — although for different reasons across different polities and time periods. Take, for example, the passage of Medicare and Medicaid in the US in 1965, following the historic triumph of the liberal wing of the Democratic Party (23), or the social democratic moment that ushered in universal health insurance in the Canadian provinces (24). In European cases, there is evidence that strong labour representation and prolonged socialist party governance has led to more expansive social programs and more robust resistance to retrenchment over time (25).

Political coalitions in favour of primary care reforms have generally not been robust enough to sustain the implementation of reform in the Canadian experience. Part of the problem lies in the way that political parties calculate the anticipated short-term effect on voter preference versus the long-run effects of policy change. Because primary care reform has been a slow-growth type of initiative, its implementation has also been plagued by the start-stop nature of party politics; in Ontario, for example, Community Health Centres have been in quasi-pilot form since the 1970s, subject to the political funding decisions of subsequent governments (26).

For a good part of the history of the development of heath care in Canada, primary care has been unable to find a strong voice, since the diffuse benefits that could be obtained were confronted with concentrated interests that, while not overtly hostile in all cases, have nevertheless been reluctant to embrace change.

How Does Change Happen in the Political System? Institutions, State Capacities and Policy Legacies

The strategies and relative success of interest organizations depend on the political system in which they operate, a system defined by the "rules of the game" that impose constraints and open opportunities to different voices (27); these rules also shape political institutions and the actors that inhabit them. We know, for example, that the division of powers in federalism can dampen program development because of the difficulties of coordinated decision making and the divided "political will" for leadership in health reform, although in some cases subnational autonomy has led to remarkable policy innovation (28). In the case of primary care the potential for such diverse innovation and policy learning is extensive. It is clear that primary care reform adapts best and can be implemented more quickly where regional health authorities already exist in the Canadian provinces (29) but change may be facilitated even in unitary systems that encourage coordination closer to the grass roots (30).

The problematic aspects of federalism have to do with cost concerns; namely, the extent to which stable funding can help underwrite some of the adjustment costs of primary care reform. But, if the February 2003 Health Accord is an example, the federal-provincial dynamic may also be affected by the federal government's use of its spending lever to encourage — and enable — provincial governments to implement primary care reform strategies. Obviously, the type of federalism also matters: even though Australia is a federal system, for example, primary care reform has been spearheaded by a consensus effort between physicians' groups and the central government, including the current efforts at amalgamating traditional general practice with integrated and geographically based "Divisions of General Practice" (31).

We also know that the size and intensity of veto points in legislative settings has a significant impact on policy outcomes, so that a consensual parliamentary system is better suited to legislating bold policy reform than a presidential system based on separation of powers (32). Nevertheless, sometimes such centralized power in the health care sector — whether in the UK or even in a federal system like that of Australia — can lead to confusion and incoherence; rapid policy reforms and changes in them have led to a certain vertigo in health reform. In Canada, parliamentary rules facilitated the legislation of bold change in the post-war era (33). Since then, the initial contours of this legislation have remained relatively stable.

Part of the institutional puzzle has to do with the way in which policy-makers and bureaucrats work within the limits of state capacity, in terms of resources and expertise, to develop and implement effective social policies (34). At the level of policy emergence, ideas are often shaped into policy through bureaucrats and the expertise they develop over time or the experts they consult through research and knowledge exchange (35). Although bureaucrats engage in "policy learning" — from the baggage they bring with them, from exchange with each other, or from policies elsewhere (36) — they function within institutions that are resistant to change. Much of the resistance comes from the way in which "learning effects" can cost valuable resources in terms of start-up costs and adaptation (37). Within the health care sector, change is also affected by the "opaque curtains" of vertical barriers to the coordination of services (38).

Recent Canadian examples reflect this type of dynamic, particularly in the case of primary care reform: within bureaucracies, innovative change models "face uphill fights" when they require extensive structural reconfigurations. Often, these barriers are reinforced by combining forces with stakeholders who may also be exposed to these types of learning costs, even though these same stakeholders may also be courted in the search for change coalitions (39).

The historical development and institutionalization of existing policies can also create living legacies that constrain policy-makers' responses. In this feedback process, breakthrough policies lead to health care systems that are bound by certain "logics" that narrow the range of feasible choices (40). Such "path dependent" development leads to a situation where politicians may be loathe to pay the political price associated with change, while at the same time, movement toward organizational change may be thwarted by the locking in of bureaucratic structures and provider interests (41).

Theories of linear change in organizations also resemble path dependency scenarios: how change leads to freeze and subsequent change occurs largely at the margins of this frozen landscape. Other models of organizational change, however, emphasize how dramatic change can occur when it is externally driven by bold movers able to build coordination and commitment from diverse players (42).

The link between policy legacies and primary care reform has been suggested by Hutchison, Abelson and Lavis (8) who argue that even "good ideas" like primary care can be stymied in the face of such barriers. What explains the magic of this Cinderella's transformation? And is this magic to be thwarted by the implementation stage of policy change?

IMPLEMENTATION, POLICIES, AND POLITICS IN PRIMARY CARE: OR, WHAT KIND OF MAGIC TRANSFORMS CINDERELLA?

In his examination of foiled attempts at national health insurance in the United States, Jonathan Oberlander asks, "why do bad things happen to good plans?" (43). As has been the case in the American experience, "desirable" health reform measures are often the least politically feasible to achieve. In fact, Oberlander argues, change will occur when the incrementalism of the status quo is no longer sustainable; in other words, when the present system breaks down in both cost control and coverage at a crisis point.

In the case of primary care in Canada, it could be argued that a convergence of cost control and access concerns had reached a crisis point — at least in the public's perception. In the past decade, major restructuring in the hospital sector across the Canadian provinces has led to changing patterns in the way Canadians access care. It has become clear, as emergency rooms overcrowd and waiting lists for elective procedures grow longer, that a new outlet for this excess demand needs to be considered. Thus, the long-simmering agenda for community-based primary care has been able to rise to the top of the "policy soup" as a feasible alternative. The interests of committed backers of primary care thus converged with state officials searching for alternative — and ostensibly lower-cost — methods of providing health care. This is true even in Quebec, where primary care has long been considered a centrepiece of the designs for integrated health and social services delivery and is now receiving renewed attention in the search for meaningful progress in health reform.

There is ample discussion in the policy literature of this type of phenomenon: how problems become priorities, policy alternatives compete, and political climates determine whether or not a policy choice gathers currency. However, there is surprisingly less attention paid to the implementation phase in the politics of health care reform. Implementation problems are usually defined as "slippage" between lawmakers' intentions and program administration (44). But implementation is more than that: it is a highly charged political phase that takes place in the "real world, with its multitude of powers, authorities and organizations, and therefore is inevitably a struggle" (45). Relatively underestimated by political scientists, "(i)mplementation is worth studying precisely because it is a struggle over the realization of ideas"; it is also best seen as an evolutionary process continuously finetuned for effectiveness (46). In other words, implementation leads to the policy legacies that feed back into the political environment and subsequent policy cycles.

The blockage in primary care reform to date is showing some opening for change. All the political signals suggest movement toward primary care reform in Canada, and most provinces have legislated or are considering legislation to create new primary care delivery structures, at least in pilot form. It has become an idea whose time has come or almost an accepted norm of health reform, at least among experts and political leaders. This has been bolstered by the newly charged sense of urgency around public health issues, the strong — and practically unanimous — voices of provincial health care reform commissions and their national counterparts, and the determination to deploy a National Health Council to monitor the progress and effects of health care reform in the provinces.

Will the implementation stage prove problematic for primary care reform? Implementation involves strong alliances and considerable commitment from groups with diverse and often conflicting objectives. Unlike the US scenarios, where strategic alliances have to be formed at the legislative stage, in Canada, policies can emerge or be legislated without such alliances, or in spite of opposing alliances. Such alliances, which at some level have to be consensual, must exist for implementation to be successful. Again in comparison to the US, the "political will" to legislate is also not enough: the passage of legislation, while contested, can be achieved in relatively short order by a majority government in a parliamentary setting. Political will cannot be a substitute — or panacea — for the difficult bargaining and negotiation required for bureaucratic and stakeholder commitment at the level of implementation. A "tipping point" for change may occur in the next few years that could wear down obstacles to change. This may be sharpened by the breakdown in incrementalism, as suggested above, or be the result of changes in pressure points from both the inside (bureaucratic politics) and outside (key interests and their voices).

As primary care moves forward onto policy agendas in the Canadian provinces, a key feature of its success will thus depend on the extent to which implementation of this reform is carried through. In other words, the real transformation of this Cinderella depends on sustaining the magic well past midnight and the end of the party, into the real life deployment of primary care reform in the health care system.

REFERENCES

1   Macinko J, Starfield B, Shi L. The contribution of primary care systems to health outcomes within OECD countries, 1970-1998. Health Services Research 2003; 38(3):831–865.

2   Hall JJ, Taylor R. Health for all beyond 2000: the demise of the Alma Ata Declaratiion and primary health care in developing countries. Medical Journal of Australia 2003;178(1):17–20.

3   Okma K. What is the best private-public model for Canadian health care? Policy Matters 2002;3(6):1–60.

4   Armstrong H, Armstrong P. Primary health care reform: A discussion paper. Ottawa: Canadian Health Coalition; 2001. Available at http://www.healthcoalition.ca/health_index.html

5   Taylor MG. Health insurance and Canadian public policy: the seven decisions that created the Canadian health insurance system and their outcomes. Second edition. Montreal: McGill-Queen's University Press; 1987.

6   Lavis J. Political elites and their influence on health-care reform in Canada. Ottawa: Commission on the Future of Health Care in Canada; 2002.

7   Naylor CD. Private practice, public payment: Canadian medicine and the politics of health insurance, 1911–1966. Montreal: McGill-Queen's University Press; 1986.

8   Hutchison B, Abelson J, Lavis J. Primary care in Canada: so much innovation, so little change. Health Affairs 2001;20(3):116–131.

9   Canadian Institute for Health Information. Health care in Canada 2003. Ottawa: the Institute; 2003.

10   White D. La santé et les services sociaux: réforme et remise en question. In: Daigle G, Rocher G, editors. Le Québec en jeu: comprendre les grands défis. Montreal: Les pressses de l'Université de Montréal; 1999. p 225–247.

11   Turgeon J, Lemieux V. La decentralisation: panacée ou boite de Pandare? In: Bégin C, Bergeron P, Forest PG, Lemieux V, editors. Le Système de santé québécois: un modèle en transformation. Montreal: Les pressses de l'Université de Montréal; 1999, p 173–194.

12   Renaud M. Réforme ou illusion? Une analyse des interventions de l'Etat québécois dans le domaine de la santé. Sociologie et Sociétés 1977; 9(1):127–152.

13   Bergeron P. La Commission Rochon reproduit les solutions de Castonguay-Nepveu. Recherches sociographiques 1990;31(3):359–380.

14   Esping-Andersen G. After the golden age? Welfare state dilemmas in a global economy. In Esping-Andersen G, editor. Welfare states in transition: national adaptations in global economies. London: Sage; 1996.

15   Pierson P. Irresistible forces, immovable objects: postindustrial welfare states confront permanent austerity. Journal of European Public Policy 1998; 5(4):539–560.

16   Butler P. Health reforms stalled by cash crisis. *The Guardian* 2003; June 3.

17   Olson M. The logic of collective action: public goods and the theory of groups. Cambridge: Harvard University Press; 1965.

18   Nathanson CA. Social movements as catalysts for policy change: the case of smoking and guns. Journal of Health Politics, Policy and Law 1999;24(3):421–488.

19   Kingdon J. Agendas, alternatives and public policies. New York: Harper Collins; 1995.

20   Martin P, Maioni A. Is the public health care model politically sustainable? Some evidence from public opinion. Proceedings of the Canadian Political Science Association, 2001:1–23.

21   Wilsford D. Doctors and the state: the politics of health care in France and the United States. Durham: Duke University Press; 1991.

22   Kelly D. Romanow, Kirby and reform of primary medical care. Healthcare Papers 2002;3(4):73–78.

23   Marmor TR. The politics of medicare. Second edition. New York: Basic Books; 2000.

24   Maioni A, Parting at the crossroads: the development of health insurance in Canada and the United States, 1940–1965. Comparative Politics 1997; 29(4):411–431.

25   Huber E, Stephens JD. Development and crisis of the welfare state: parties and policies in global markets. Chicago: University of Chicago Press; 2001.

26   Suschnigg C. Reforming Ontario's primary health care system: one step forward, two steps back? International Journal of Health Services 2001;31(1):91–103.

27   March J, Olsen J. The new institutionalism: organizational factors in political life. American Political Science Review 1984;3(9):734–749.

28   Corbett S, Banting KG. Multi-level governance and health care: health policy in five federations. In Banting KG, Corbett S. Health policy and federalism. A comparative perspective. Kingston: Institute of Intergovernmental Relations at Queen's University; 2002.

29   Doctor Sadok Besrour Chair in Family Medicine of the University of Montreal. The team in primary care: a new vision, new ways to work. Montreal: The Chair; 2002.

30   Brown LD. Comparing health systems in four countries: lessons for the United States. American Journal of Public Health 2003;93(1):52–56.

31   Russell G. Primary care reform: view from Australia. Canadian Family Physician 2002;48(3):440–443.

32   Immergut EM. Health politics: interests and institutions in Western Europe. Cambridge: Cambridge University Press; 1992.

33   Maioni A. Parting at the crossroads: the emergence of health insurance in the United States and Canada. Princeton: Princeton University Press; 1998.

34   Weir M and Skocpol T. State structures and the possibilities for "Keynesian" responses to the Great Depression in Sweden, Britain, and the United States. In Evans PB,

Rueschemeyer R, Skocpol T. Bringing the state back in. Princeton: Princeton University Press; 1985.

35   Lavis JN, Ross SE, Stoddart GL, Hohenadel JM, McLeod CB, Evans RG. Do Canadian civil servants care about the health of populations? American Journal of Public Health 2003;93(4):658–663.

36   Heclo H. Modern social politics in Britain and Sweden; from relief to income maintenance. New Haven: Yale University Press; 1974.

37   North DC. Institutions, institutional change, and economic performance. Cambridge: Cambridge University Press; 1990.

38   Glouberman S, Mintzberg H. Managing the care of health and the cure of disease—part II: integration. Health Care Management Review 2001;26(1):70–84.

39   Marriott J, Mable AL. An overview of progress and potential in health system integration in Canada. Health Services Division, Health Canada, November 2002.

40   Tuohy CH. Accidental logics: the dynamics of change in the health care arena. New York: Oxford University Press; 1999.

41   Pierson P. When effect becomes cause: policy feedback and political change. World Politics 1993;45(4):595–628.

42   Elwyn G, Rhydderch M. Achieving organizational change in primary care: simmer gently for two years. Preventive Medicine 2002;35:419–421.

43   Oberlander J. The politics of health reform: why do bad things happen to good plans? Health Affairs Web Exclusive 2003; W3391—W3404.

44   Brooks S. Public policy in Canada: an introduction. Toronto: Oxford University Press; 1998. p 77.

45   Pal LA. Public policy analysis: an introduction. Second edition. Toronto: Nelson; 1992. p 177.

46   Majone G, Wildavsky A. Implementation as evolution. In Pressman J, Wildavsky A. Implementation. Second edition. Berkeley: University of California Press; 1979. p 194.

Primary Health Care Renewal in Canada
Are We Nearly There?

Brian Hutchison

Since the advent of Canadian medicare, efforts to reform primary care have faced formidable barriers to systemic change. Among the most fundamental of these are the policy legacies of Canada's federal/provincial division of powers, the principle of public payment for private medical practice, and the privileging of physician and hospital services in the *Canada Health Act* (1–3). Further, the ways in which Canadian policy-makers have pursued primary health care reform have themselves been obstacles to significant system-level change. Task forces, commissions, and policy-makers charged with making recommendations for improving primary care in Canada have almost always proposed the universal implementation of an "ideal" model for primary care organization and delivery (4–8). By bundling together a comprehensive set of reforms, this approach has guaranteed widespread opposition from physicians, the currently dominant primary care providers. Support for proposed models has been limited by the acceptability to stakeholders of their least attractive features.

Canadian policy-makers, analysts, and many health care stakeholders have tended to see change in funding and payment methods as a necessary condition for strengthening primary care. For example, the Premier's Advisory Council on Health for Alberta identified fee-for-service payment as "an almost insurmountable barrier to change" (9). In general, policy-makers have tended to demonize fee-for-service and glorify capitation payment methods, although the belief that capitation funding of primary care enhances quality of care, achieves cost savings, and improves efficiency is not supported — or for that matter refuted — by high quality evidence (1, 10).

Means to policy ends, such as payment methods, group practice, and multidisciplinary practice, sometimes seem to have become ends in themselves. Further, the logical and evidentiary links between policy objectives and proposed reforms have often been tenuous, providing easy ammunition to those opposed to change.

Finally, policy-makers have frequently done a poor job of anticipating the likely responses of key stakeholders to their policy initiatives. Conceptually, policy initiatives can be seen as sending messages regarding the individuals and organizations the policy initiative is intended to influence, desired behaviours, and the inducements on offer (11). Failure to anticipate and address the potential responses of stakeholders that could compromise the achievement of policy goals is clearly evident in the history of Ontario's Health Service Organization Program (12) and in the recurring failure of proposals for radical system-wide change in primary health care.

Flawed approaches to the development and implementation of primary health care policy — especially the pursuit of sweeping changes in the face of unfavourable circumstances — have left the basic structure of primary care organization, funding, and delivery intact and resulted in missed opportunities for cumulative incremental change at the system level (1).

A NEW POLICY ENVIRONMENT?

Despite this seemingly gloomy picture, during the past several years Canadian policy-makers appear to have absorbed a number of key lessons from the gridlock of the last three decades, as evidenced by recent provincial reports (9,13). The first of these lessons is that there is no single "right" model for the funding, organization, and delivery of primary health care. Different models have different strengths and limitations. Some serve particular populations especially well. Most are capable of evolutionary development. And some models are potentially complementary. Second, neither capitation nor any other particular funding or payment method holds the key to primary care transformation. Third, the policy-making slate is anything but clean. The future of primary health care must acknowledge the past and be achievable starting from the present. Fourth, change requires resources. Primary health care renewal will incur substantial costs and require major investments in primary care infrastructure.

Key features of the current policy environment include a new-found willingness of provincial, territorial, and federal governments, as health system funders, to invest in primary health care infrastructure. The recommendations of the Romanow Commission and their reflection in the First Minister's Health Care Accord offer the promise of substantial resources specifically designated to support primary health care renewal. They also place a heavy onus on the federal and provincial governments, and indirectly on regional health authorities, to deliver tangible improvements in primary care access and quality.

Policy-makers have begun to show a growing tolerance for pluralism of organizational and funding models and an increasing acceptance of incremental approaches to systemic change (9,13). For their part, both physicians and the public demonstrate an increasing openness to change. For example, only one-third of primary care physicians responding to the Canadian Medical Association's 2003 Physician Resource Questionnaire identified fee-for-service as their preferred method of payment (14). In a 1999 survey of members of the Ontario College of Family Physicians, 70 percent indicated they would welcome the opportunity to work collaboratively with publicly funded nurse practitioners (15). The Ontario College has strongly supported the province's Family Health Network (FHN) program, while proposing enhancements to the FHN model and stressing the importance of voluntary participation and physician choice of organizational models and remuneration methods (16). Among respondents to the Medical Post's 2001 National Survey of Doctors, 42 percent indicated that doctors should "relinquish some power/responsibility to other health care professionals such as nurse practitioners" (17). As a reflection of changing public attitudes, 77 percent of respondents to the Fall/Winter 2002 HealthInsider Survey said they would be willing to see a nurse practitioner instead of a doctor "for minor illnesses such as colds, sore throats, allergies, etc." and 76 percent would see a nurse practitioner for support and advice on maintaining their health (18).

This new policy environment opens up possibilities for significant system level change that is incremental, cumulative, and allows for multiple complementary and continually evolving organizational and funding models. Unbundling the components of primary care models would allow early, system-wide implementation of those elements with broad public and stakeholder support. Pluralism of models offers opportunities to those ready to embrace innovation, without attempting to impose change on the remainder.

IMPLEMENTING PRIMARY HEALTH CARE RENEWAL

Proposals for primary health care renewal in Canada have included varying mixtures of the following elements: patient registration with a primary care provider, group practice, multidisciplinary practice, alternatives to fee-for-service remuneration, information management systems, mechanisms for coordination of care, quality improvement mechanisms, and defined service standards and accountability arrangements. If, as we have suggested elsewhere (1), the components of recently proposed models of primary care are largely divisible and capable of independent implementation, an assessment of factors in the policy environment that either facilitate or impede the implementation of individual components becomes highly relevant for policy-making. Facilitators and barriers related to commonly suggested primary care reform elements are summarized in Table 1 and described below.

Patient Registration with a Primary Care Provider

In exchange for some restriction on their ability to simultaneously use multiple sources of primary care, registered patients receive assured access to a defined range of health care services under specified terms and conditions from a provider who makes an explicit commitment to coordinate and monitor their health care. By identifying the population served by a provider, patient registration provides the foundation for an effective, responsive, and accountable system of primary health care. A patient list is fundamental to understanding the burden of illness in a population as the basis for planning both anticipatory and responsive services, especially preventive care and chronic disease management.

Ninety-two percent of respondents to the national Spring/Summer 2001 HealthInsider telephone survey — up from 83 percent in 1997 and 86 percent in 1999 — approved of a relationship in which they would register with one "regular or family doctor" who would ensure that they and their family would receive all necessary medical services and arrange for medical specialists and other health services as needed (19). Experience from Ontario's primary care reform pilots indicates that only a tiny minority of patients decline registration (20).

Barriers to the implementation of patient registration include a lack of evidence that registration per se leads to improvements in quality of care and accountability, potential public concern about limitations on choice of provider, and the resources (including provider time) required to introduce and maintain patient registration. In a survey of Hamilton physicians participating in Ontario's primary care reform pilot project, 19.2 percent identified the patient registration process as a challenge or problem, second only to information technology which was identified as a challenge by 20.8 percent of respondents (20).

TABLE 1

IMPLEMENTING COMPONENTS OF PRIMARY CARE REFORM

Component	Facilitators	Barriers
Patient registration	• Enables proactive approaches to preventive care and chronic disease management • Supports population-based planning of services and programs at the practice level • Facilitates coordination of care • Substantial public support	• Resources (including provider time) required to introduce and maintain patient registration • Potential public concern about limitations on choice of provider • Lack of evidence that registration per se improves quality of care
Group practice	• Builds on a continuing trend • Offers the possibility of improved working conditions for providers • Substantial professional and public support	• Professional medical culture based on individual clinical autonomy and control over practice organization • Costs associated with the transition to group practice • Increased requirements for infrastructure and administration
Multidisciplinary practice	• Shortage of primary care physicians • Increasing physician workloads • Increasing physician exposure during training to multi-disciplinary primary health care teams • Growing support among primary care physicians for collaborative interdisciplinary practice • Public openness to team-based primary health care	• Capital and ongoing overhead costs associated with adding new disciplines to existing practices • Perceived threat to physicians' scope of practice and physician-patient relationships
Alternatives to fee-for-service remuneration	• Declining allegiance to fee-for-service among primary care physicians • Growing willingness of policy-makers to entertain blended payment schemes	• Policy-makers' continuing enchantment with capitation payment • Alternatives to fee-for-service perceived by some primary care physicians as a threat to clinical autonomy

... continued

TABLE 1
CONT'D.

Component	Facilitators	Barriers
Information management systems	• Appeal to providers' motivations to deliver high quality care • Substantial public and professional support for electronic health records	• Costs of development, implementation and maintenance • Investments of provider time and effort required for startup and maintenance • Disappointingly limited impact to date on clinical care and practice-level decision making
Mechanisms for coordination/ integration of care	• Widespread recognition of deficiencies • Considerable professional and public support for information sharing	• Perceived threat of formal integration to physician autonomy and continuity of patient-provider relationships • Potential for integration to divert resources from clinical service to administrative functions
Quality improvement mechanisms	• Appeal to providers' commitment to high quality care • Support of physicians' organizations for enhanced quality improvement • Accumulating evidence in support of specific quality improvement methods	• Provider anxieties about scrutiny by peers and managers • Logistical challenges of mounting collaborative quality improvement programs • Need for financial, organizational, and technical support
Defined service standards and accountability arrangements	• Strong *prima facie* case • Growing support among physicians' organizations for defined service standards • Increasing precedents for contractual arrangements between primary care providers and health system funders/ managers	• Tradition of professional self-governance • Medicare's "founding bargain" of public payment for private practice between physicians and the state

Group Practice

Efforts to promote group practice have the advantage of building on a well-established trend; among respondents to the Canadian Medical Association's Physician Resource Questionnaire, the proportion of primary care physicians who report being in solo practice has fallen from 33 percent in 1998 to 18.4 percent in 2003 (21,22). Group practices and practice networks are favoured by influential physician organizations such as the College of Family Physicians of Canada and the Ontario College of Family Physicians (23,24,25). In a Canada Health Monitor national telephone survey carried out between December 1995 and January 1996, 64 percent of respondents strongly approved (24 percent) or somewhat approved (40 percent) of group practice arrangements even if they would not see their regular doctor (26). Group practice offers the possibility of improved working conditions for primary care physicians through greater availability of coverage for vacations and time off and increased sharing of on-call responsibilities. As a function of scale, larger group practices have potential advantages with respect to the development of clinical information systems, quality improvement activities, and use of non-physician health professionals.

Impediments to the spread of group practice include a professional culture based on individual clinical autonomy and control over practice organization, costs associated with the transition to group practice, and increased requirements for infrastructure and administration. Evidence regarding the relationship between group practice and quality of care is mixed (27). Three Canadian studies, two conducted in Ontario and one in Manitoba, have shown no independent association between group (vs solo) practice and quality of care (28,29). Another Ontario study found that, after controlling for other factors, solo family physicians provided higher quality preventive care to unannounced standardized patients than group practice physicians (30).

Multidisciplinary Practice

Factors favouring the development of multidisciplinary practice include a shortage of primary care providers, rising physician workloads, increasing exposure during training to multidisciplinary primary health care delivery, and growing openness among primary care physicians and the public to interdisciplinary practice. Since the late 1990s, a growing consensus has formed among health care providers, policy-makers, and the public that Canada faces a significant and growing shortage of primary care physicians. Rather than protecting turf, many primary care physicians are looking for people to share it.

Primary care physicians are an increasingly unhappy lot. A report by the
Ontario College of Family Physicians on the working conditions of family
doctors was tellingly subtitled "Too many hours, too much stress, too little
respect" (31). A recent *Toronto Star* story on the changing work life and expectations of family physicians carried the headlines "Family medicine has
become exhausting" and "Money can't compensate for time with your family"
(32). Respondents to the Canadian Medical Association's 2001 Physician Resource Questionnaire complained of heavy workloads and negative effects of
career on family and personal life (33).

Mainstream physician organizations are beginning to express support,
albeit cautious, for collaborative primary care practice models (24,25,34,35).
The College of Family Physicians of Canada envisions networked family physicians who "would work together with nurses and other health care
professionals as part of the family practice network team" (24).

The Canadian Policy Research Network conducted a Citizens' Dialogue
on the Future of Health Care in Canada for the Romanow Commission on the
Future of Health Care in Canada (36). Twelve day-long dialogue sessions were
held across Canada between January and March of 2002 with citizens who had
been randomly selected to provide a representative cross-section of the Canadian population. When prompted to consider health system reforms, the
participants "[saw] the potential in having a team of medical professionals
(doctors, nurses, pharmacists and others) to provide more coordinated primary
care... They also [were] very attracted by the idea that such a team would not
only provide more coordinated, cost-effective care, but also would have greater
incentive to focus on wellness, prevention and patient education..." The report
from this consultation exercise concluded that "Canadians expect responsive
team-based care, led by doctors." By way of caution, it should be noted how
the consideration of primary care reorganization was framed. Participants were
asked to respond to the following scenario: "Reorganize service delivery in
order to provide more integrated care, realize efficiencies and expand coverage. Each Canadian would sign up with a health care provider network who
would work as a team to provide more coordinated, cost-effective services and
improved access to care." Facilitators prompted discussion of specific primary
care reform options with the question, "To reduce cost and improve efficiency,
are we prepared to... ?" Framing the discussion in this way incorporates the
untested assumption that these innovations in primary health care delivery would
result in improved access, coordination, and efficiency.

In his analysis of public opinion research on the health care system since
1985, Mendelsohn (37) makes the following assessment regarding Canadians'
views on primary health care teams: "In general, there appears to be a good

deal of openness to the idea of primary health service teams, although Canadians have not yet thought much about the issue. Canadians might oppose a change that threatened their relationship with their family physician, although there are no reliable data on this precise question. The overwhelming majority of Canadians continue to have a family physician and any move to the implementation of health service teams would need to allow Canadians to choose their own family doctor and develop the level of trust that comes with such a relationship."

Barriers to the implementation of multidisciplinary practice include capital and ongoing overhead costs associated with adding new disciplines to existing practices (16) and a perceived threat to physicians' scope of practice and physician-patient relationships (38).

Alternatives to Fee-for-Service Remuneration

Strategically, primary health care policy-makers, analysts, and many health care stakeholders have focused their attention on funding and remuneration methods as the key to primary health care renewal. The consideration of options generally centres on the incentive structures associated with each of the existing and alternative funding and payment mechanisms. Fee-for-service, the currently dominant mode of physician remuneration in Canada, rewards productivity but encourages the provision of services by physicians rather than other equally or better qualified providers and rewards the provision of service irrespective of need. Capitation focuses attention on the health needs of a practice population and allows flexible use of health care personnel, but rewards withholding service (stinting on care), off-loading primary care to specialists, and "cream skimming" (also referred to as "cherry picking"). Salary payment allows providers to allocate time and effort to yield maximum health benefits, but also rewards "being there" regardless of productivity. Under what conditions and to what extent health organizations and providers respond to these incentives are unanswered questions.

Current conditions favourable to the uptake of alternative payment mechanisms include declining allegiance to fee-for-service payment among primary care physicians and the growing willingness of policy-makers to entertain blended payment schemes. Among family physicians/general practitioners who responded to the Canadian Medical Association's 2003 Physician Resource Questionnaire, 34.8 percent identified fee-for-service as their preferred payment method; 35.7 percent preferred some form of time-based payment (salary or sessional/hourly payment); 21 percent preferred blended payment and 1.3 percent preferred capitation (14). Among respondents to the 2001 Physician

Resource Questionnaire who preferred blended payment, only 3 percent specified capitation as a desirable component of blended payment in their open-ended responses (Canadian Medical Association/McMaster Centre for Health Economics and Policy Analysis, unpublished data; 2003).

In response to primary care physicians' aversion to capitation payment and a growing belief that targeted payments may be useful mechanisms for encouraging the provision of services aligned with health system needs, policy-makers have shown increasing willingness to negotiate blended payment schemes. For example, the Ontario Family Network (FHN) blended payment model includes age and sex adjusted capitation payments, fee-for-service, and a variety of targeted payments. FHN physicians who choose the blended payment option receive 10 percent of the value of fee-for-service claims for included (core) services and can bill fee-for-service for excluded (non-core) services and for services provided to non-enrolled patients.

Barriers to the adoption of alternative physician remuneration methods include policy-makers' continuing enchantment with capitation and the perception of many physicians that alternatives to fee-for-service threaten clinical autonomy, in part because they usually involve a contractual relationship between the physician or provider organization and the ministry of health or regional health authority. From a health system manager's perspective, capitation has several virtues. First, it delegates responsibility for ensuring access to appropriate health services to the capitated provider. Second, health care expenditures under capitation are controllable and predictable. Third, it avoids the incentive to "overservice" (and hence increase health care costs) inherent in fee-for-service remuneration. Fourth, capitation funding allows health care providers to meet patients' needs in the most appropriate and efficient fashion because payments are not tied, as with fee-for-service, to delivery of services by physicians. However, capitation could be more or less costly and more or less efficient than alternative funding/payment methods, depending on the level of capitation payments and the conditions under which capitation is implemented. For example, under current conditions of unmet need for primary care services due to shortages of providers, conversion from fee-for-service to capitation, in the absence of available physician substitutes such as nurse practitioners, might be harmful given the incentive to limit service provision under capitation. Whereas fee-for-service physicians might be inclined to increase the volume of services they provide in response to patient demand, capitated providers might be less likely to do so. On the other hand, the effects of a change from fee-for-service to capitation might be more sanguine under conditions of provider surplus.

Information Management Systems

Clinically focused information management systems appeal to providers' motivations to deliver high quality care and are championed by influential professional organizations (16,18,19). Among Canadians polled in the Health Care in Canada Survey 2002, 69 percent agreed (28 percent strongly) with "implementing electronic patient records to improve the integration of services and monitor the use of health care resources, even if this means that patient health information may be accessible by other health care providers" (39). Among health care providers, support was even stronger, at 73 percent of doctors, 76 percent of nurses, 85 percent of pharmacists, and 86 percent of health care managers.

Factors that militate against the diffusion of sophisticated and clinically useful information management systems include the costs of system development, implementation and maintenance, and the substantial investments of provider time and effort that are required for system startup and maintenance. Provider enthusiasm for committing the required time and energy may be dampened by the disappointingly limited impact to date of existing information management systems on clinical care and practice-level decision making.

Mechanisms for Coordination of Care

Canada's health care system is frequently described as lacking in mechanisms to promote coordination and integration, resulting in fragmentation of care and duplication of effort (8, 40–44). Possible approaches to enhancing coordination include regulations that define standards for communication between: (i) the primary health care provider making a referral and the person or agency to whom the patient is referred; (ii) first-contact health care providers serving patients in common (e.g., family physicians, nurse practitioners, optometrists, physiotherapists, public health nurses, midwives, emergency rooms, home care programs, chiropractors, long-term care facilities); and (iii) health care providers in other sectors such as education, housing, and social services. An example of this approach is Ontario's requirement for a referral letter from the primary care physician for a specialist physician to bill a consultation fee. This requirement not only promotes communication but also discourages direct patient access to secondary care. Mechanisms to promote access to specialist services on a referral-only basis help to establish the primary care provider in a coordinating, facilitating, and advocacy role. The primary health care provider's task includes "help[ing] patients to avoid inappropriate entry to the pipelines of secondary care — not because these are costly but because they waste everybody's time, incur unnecessary risks and divert attention for more relevant and effective solutions" (45).

Information technology that permits sharing of information based on electronic health records among health care providers is frequently advanced as a means of enhancing communication and coordination of care (24,25). In the National Health Care in Canada Survey 2001, two-thirds or more of the public, doctors, nurses, pharmacists, and health care managers felt that care should be coordinated across the health care system "all the time," although one-third or less thought this was happening now (46).

Calls for improved coordination and service integration are common to many proposals for primary care renewal and health system reform (7–9,40,41,43,47). Existing or proposed models for integration range from informal networking at the practice/organization level and forums for discussion and joint planning at the inter-organizational, community or regional levels, to health care organizations that are fully integrated both horizontally (across primary care, community care, long-term care, and sometimes public health and social services) and vertically (primary, secondary, tertiary, and quaternary health care services). Physician organizations have only recently begun to address the issue of integration in position papers on primary care renewal (16,25). Formal integration runs contrary to the tradition of independent, clinically autonomous, physician-owned and managed, solo and small group practices and raises the spectre of organizational complexity, increased administrative and transactions costs, diffusion of responsibility, and diseconomies of scale.

Quality Improvement Mechanisms

Quality improvement programs appeal to health care providers' commitment to high quality care. The need to develop effective quality improvement mechanisms is widely acknowledged by physician organizations (16,25,48). There is growing evidence that quality improvement activities involving methods such as standard-setting, patient and provider reminder systems, use of practice facilitators, and audit and feedback are of value in improving processes and outcomes of care (49–56).

Barriers to the implementation of continuous quality improvement mechanisms in primary health care include provider anxieties about scrutiny by peers and health system managers. These concerns can be addressed, at least in part, by ensuring that quality improvement activities are peer led and by maintaining a clear separation between quality improvement and performance monitoring. Julian Tudor Hart has eloquently cautioned against linking practice audit in aid of quality improvement with rewards for "good" performance: "Information technology... makes mass clinical audit possible so that practice in whole populations can for the first time become routinely self-critical, and care can begin to merge with science. This requires that audit data be used only to discover the truth, not to reward or punish competing entrepreneurs whose incomes depend on data they record" (45).

Other barriers to the widespread implementation of quality improvement in primary care include the logistical challenges of mounting collaborative quality improvement programs in the context of small group practices or practice networks and the heavy clinical service demands currently faced by primary care providers. Because few primary health care providers have either the training or access to technical support (not to speak of time) required to carry out effective quality improvement activities, substantial financial, organizational, and technical support will be necessary.

Defined Service Standards and Accountability Arrangements

The *prima facie* case for defined service standards and accountability mechanisms is strong: health care providers who are paid from the public purse should be accountable to the regional health authority or provincial government (as health care funder and system manager) for providing services of acceptable quality under defined terms and conditions. However, clinical accountability to government or a government agency defies the tradition of professional self-governance and can be seen as violating the founding bargain between the medical profession and government on which medicare is based — an accommodation that allowed for the continuation of physicians' clinical autonomy and control over the location and organization of medical practice (2).

Notwithstanding this conflict, there appears to be growing support among physician organizations for service standards that include a defined "basket" of comprehensive primary care services and the availability of some form of urgent care response 24 hours a day, 7 days a week (16,23,25). Alternative payment plans for primary care providers usually involve a contractual agreement that defines service standards. In Ontario, contracts between the Ministry of Health and Long-Term Care and Health Service Organizations, Primary Care Networks, Family Health Networks and Family Health Groups specify minimum numbers of office hours per week, 24/7 on-call availability, and a defined basket of services. However, both the fact and the complexity of these contracts have been thought to deter physician participation in alternative funding arrangements.

Clearly, a variety of accountability arrangements is possible. For example, the Ontario College of Family Physicians has suggested an accountability framework that includes an accreditation process, measurement of performance against provincially and locally defined outcome expectations, and community advisory committees that would oversee "accountability measurement" and provide feedback to practice networks, coordinate their activities and facilitate integration with the broader health care system (16).

PUTTING THE PIECES TOGETHER

Pursuing the implementation of individual components of primary health care renewal at different paces and with different (but overlapping) groups of primary care providers and organizations is not a risk-free change strategy. Potential pitfalls of an incremental and pluralistic approach to primary care renewal include a lack of system coherence, high administrative and transaction costs associated with multiple organizational and funding models, and a change process that can become bogged down in the details of implementing a variety of reform elements independently (1). However, in a policy environment that continues to offer unfavourable conditions for rapid, fundamental change, these risks need to be balanced against the alternative, which has, for the last three decades, been policy gridlock.

By articulating a clear sense of policy direction, policy-makers can help to avoid some of these pitfalls. Outlining the anticipated future shape of primary health care (including its relationship to other sectors) and indicating the way in which existing primary care models are expected to evolve may prevent policy-makers, health care managers, and professional leaders from losing sight of longer term objectives and help allay the anxieties of stakeholders about "hidden agendas." The policy destination need not be a single universal model, but could be a primary health care system based on complementary and interdependent models. By the same token, the roadmap to renewal could offer alternative routes. Priorities for primary health care innovations might be guided by considerations such as: consistency with health system objectives, quality and strength of evidence of effectiveness, acceptability to key stakeholders and the public, availability of required resources, and availability or potential to develop needed technology.

Given the paucity of available evidence regarding the impact of existing and proposed primary health care models and many suggested model components, innovations in primary health care should be subjected to thoughtful and rigorous evaluation as a matter of course. Evaluation should address both implementation and impact, so that shortcomings can be identified and overcome and successes reinforced and disseminated.

Returning to my original question, "Primary health care renewal: Are we nearly there?" — the answer appears to be "no," but the journey has begun.

REFERENCES

1   Hutchison B, Abelson J, Lavis J. Primary care in Canada: so much innovation, so little change. Health Affairs 2001;20(3):116–131.

2   Tuohy CH. Accidental logics: the dynamics of change in the health care arena in the United States, Britain, and Canada. New York: Oxford University Press; 1999.

3   Hacker JS. The historical logic of national health insurance: structure and sequence in the development of British, Canadian, and US medical policy. Studies in American Political Development 1998;(Spring):57–103.

4   Hastings JEF. The Community Health Centre in Canada. Ottawa: Information Canada; 1973.

5   Federal/Provincial/Territorial Advisory Committee on Health Services. The Victoria report on physician remuneration: a model for the reorganization of primary care and the introduction of population-based funding, a discussion document. Victoria: the Advisory Committee; July 1995.

6   National Forum on Health. Canada health action: building on the legacy — final report. Ottawa: National Forum on Health; 1997.

7   Health Services Restructuring Commission. Primary health care strategy. Toronto: the Commission; 1999.

8   Saskatchewan Commission on Medicare. KJ Fyke, Commissioner. Caring for medicare: sustaining a quality system. Regina: Policy and Planning Branch, Saskatchewan Health; 2001.

9   Alberta. Premier's Advisory Council on Health. D Mazankowski, Chair. Report of the Premier's Advisory Council on Health: a framework for reform. Edmonton: the Council; 2001.

10   Shortt SED. Primary care reform: is there a clinical rationale? In: Wilson R, Shortt SED, Dorland J, editors. Implementing primary care reform: barriers and facilitators. Montreal and Kingston: School of Policy Studies, Queen's University and McGill-Queen's University Press; 2004. p 11–24.

11   Giacomini M, Hurley J, Lomas J, Bhatia V, Goldsmith L. The many meanings of money: a health policy analysis framework for understanding financial incentives. Hamilton, Ontario: McMaster University Centre for Health Economics and Policy Analysis, Working Paper Series 96–6; August 1996.

12   Gillett J, Hutchison B, Birch S. Capitation and primary care in Canada: financial incentives and the evaluation of Health Service Organizations. International Journal of Health Services 2001;31(3):583–603.

13 Primary Care Advisory Committee. K LeGrow, Chair. The family physician's role in a continuum of care framework for Newfoundland and Labrador: a framework for primary care renewal. St. John's: the Committee; 2001.

14 Canadian Medical Association. Results of the CMA's 2003 Physician Resource Questionnaire. Available at http://www.cmaj.ca/cgi/data/169/7/701/DC1/26 Accessed January 26, 2004.

15 Ontario College of Family Physicians. FP survey: working with nurse practitioners. Toronto: Ontario College of Family Physicians; January 1999.

16 Ontario College of Family Physicians. Ensuring success for Ontario's Family Health Networks — leadership, innovation, accountability and connectivity in family medicine. Toronto: Ontario College of Family Physicians; June 19, 2001.

17 Medical Post. The Medical Post 2001 National Survey of Doctors. Toronto: The Medical Post; November 27, 2001, supplement. p 18.

18 IBM Business Consulting Services. Primary care. HealthInsider Survey 2002;8(Fall/Winter):19–23.

19 PricewaterhouseCoopers. Primary care. HealthInsider 2001;5(Spring-Summer):15–19.

20 Neimanis IM, Paterson JM, Allega RL. Primary care reform: physicians' participation in Hamilton-Wentworth. Canadian Family Physician 2002;48:306–313.

21 Canadian Medical Association. eCMAJ — data supplement — practice setting. Available at http://www.cmaj.ca/cgi/content/full/159/5/525/DC1/3 Accessed October 30, 2003.

22 Canadian Medical Association. Results of the CMA's 2003 Physician Resource Questionnaire. Available at http://www.cmaj.ca/cgi/data/169/7/701/DC1/23 Accessed January 26, 2004.

23 College of Family Physicians of Canada. Primary care and family medicine in Canada: a prescription for renewal. Mississauga: College of Family Physicians of Canada; October 2000.

24 College of Family Physicians of Canada. Shaping the future of health care: submission to the Commission on the Future of Health Care in Canada. Mississauga: College of Family Physicians of Canada; October 25, 2001.

25 Ontario College of Family Physicians. Family medicine in the 21st century: a prescription for excellent healthcare. Toronto: Ontario College of Family Physicians; November 30, 1999.

26 Berger E, Price Waterhouse. Canada Health Monitor. Survey 13. December 1995–1996, page 18. Toronto.

27 Donabedian A. The epidemiology of quality. Inquiry 1985;22:282–292.

28 Borgiel A, Williams JI, Bass MJ, Dunn EV, Evensen MK, Lamont CT, et al. Quality of care in family practice: does residency training make a difference? Canadian Medical Association Journal 1989;140:1035–1043.

29 Roos N. Impact of the organization of practice on quality of care and physician productivity. Medical Care 1980;18:347–359.

30 Hutchison B, Woodward CA, Norman G, Brown JA, Abelson J. Provision of preventive care to unannounced standardized patients. Canadian Medical Association Journal 1998;158:185–193.

31 Ontario College of Family Physicians. Implementation strategies: "too many hours, too much stress, too little respect." Toronto: Ontario College of Family Physicians; July 19, 2000.

32 Palmer K, Lu V. Family medicine has become exhausting. Toronto Star; June 17, 2002.

33   Canadian Medical Association. 2001 CMA Physician Resource Questionnaire Results. Available at http://www.cma.ca/cmaj/Vol-165/ISSUE-5/prq/index.asp Accessed September 4, 2001.

34   Barrett P. Presentation to the Standing Senate Committee on Social Affairs, Science and Technology. Ottawa: Canadian Medical Association; May 22, 2002.

35   Hutchison SJ. Presentation to the Standing Senate Committee on Social Affairs, Science and Technology. Ottawa: Canadian Medical Association; May 22, 2002.

36   Maxwell J, Jackson K, Legowski B, Rosell S, Yankelovich D. Report on citizens' dialogue on the future of health care in Canada. Saskatoon: Commission on the Future of Health Care in Canada; June 2002.

37   Mendelsohn M. Canadian's thoughts on their health care system: preserving the Canadian model through innovation. Saskatoon: Commission on the Future of Health Care in Canada; June 2002.

38   Ontario College of Family Physicians. Implementation strategies: protecting trust in the patient-physician relationship. Toronto: Ontario College of Family Physicians; June 19, 2000.

39   Health Care in Canada Survey. Health care in Canada Survey 2002: a national survey of health care providers, managers and the public. Toronto: Virtual Learning Inc.; 2002.

40   Health Service Restructuring Commission. A vision of Ontario's health services system. Toronto: the Commission; January 1997.

41   Leatt P, Pink GH, Guerriere M. Towards a Canadian model of integrated healthcare. Healthcare Papers 2000;1:13-35.

42   Canada. Parliament. Senate. Standing Committee on Social Affairs, Science and Technology. MJL Kirby, Chair. The health of Canadians — the federal role. Final report on the state of the health care system in Canada. Vol. 6: recommendations for reform. Ottawa: the Senate Standing Committee; 2002.

43   Commission on the Future of Health Care in Canada. RJ Romanow, Commissioner. Building on values: the future of health care in Canada — final report. Ottawa: the Commission; November 2002.

44   Rosser WW, Kasperski J. Organizing primary care for an integrated system. Healthcare Papers 1999;1(1):5-21.

45   Hart JT. Two paths for medical practice. Lancet 1992;340:772–775.

46   Health Care in Canada Survey. Health Care in Canada Survey 2001: a national survey of health care providers, managers and the public. Toronto: Virtual Learning Inc.; 2001.

47   Quebec. Study Commission on Health and Social Services. Emerging solutions: report and recommendations. Quebec: the Commission; 2001.

48   College of Family Physicians of Canada. Managing change: the family medicine group practice model. Mississauga: College of Family Physicians of Canada; 1995.

49   North of England Study of Standards and Performance in General Practice. Medical audit in general practice. I. Effects on doctors' clinical behaviour for common childhood conditions. British Medical Journal 1992;304:1480–1484.

50   North of England Study of Standards and Performance in General Practice. II. Effects on health of patients with common childhood conditions. British Medical Journal 1992;304:1484–1488.

51   Buntinx F, Winkens R, Grol R, Knottnerus JA. Influencing diagnostic and preventive performance in ambulatory care by feedback and reminders: a review. Family Practice 1993;10:219–228.

52 Davis DA, Thomson MA, Oxman AD, Haynes RB. Changing physician performance: a systematic review of the effect of continuing medical education strategies. Journal of the American Medical Association 1995;274:700–705.

53 Fullard E, Fowler F, Gray M. Promotion prevention in primary care: a controlled trial of low technology, low cost approach. British Medical Journal 1987;294:1880–1882.

54 Dietrich AJ, O'Connor GT, Keller A, Carney PA, Levy D, Whaley FS. Cancer: improving early detection and prevention. A community practice randomized trial. British Medical Journal 1992;304:687–691.

55 Jones JN, Marsden P. Improved diabetes care in a UK health district. Diabetic Medicine 1992;9:176–180.

56 Bryce FP, Neville RG, Crombie IK, Clark RA, McKenzie P. Controlled trial of an audit facilitator in diagnosis and treatment of childhood asthma in general practice. British Medical Journal 1995;310:838–842.

Implementing Primary Care Reform in Canada
Barriers and Facilitators

Cathy Fooks

INTRODUCTION

Governments and health care stakeholders have been talking about reorganizing the way Canadians receive primary care services for a very long time (1). Yet it is hard to discern real change at the local level — publicly funded medical and hospital services are organized largely the way they were at the inception of Canadian medicare. Despite solid evidence services could be organized more effectively and achieve better health outcomes for citizens, reform is slow in coming (2). Why?

This paper briefly describes the current policy directions taken by provinces in reforming their primary care services and analyzes implementation barriers and facilitators to realizing those policy directions.

DEFINITIONS

Terms abound: primary care, primary health care, primary care services, etc. A recent review of international models makes a useful distinction between primary care and primary health care (3). The authors describe primary care as the diagnosis, treatment, and management of health problems with services delivered largely by physicians. Primary health care is described as including primary care, but also including the broader determinants of health such as sickness prevention and health promotion activities that are provided by physicians and others in a team-based environment.

It is clear when looking at current provincial reforms that a variety of terms are used somewhat interchangeably:

Alberta Primary Health Care is based on a holistic definition of health that recognizes the influence of social, economic, and environmental factors on a person's well-being; is delivered by a variety of providers; and emphasizes the coordination of health services, health promotion, illness and injury prevention to cover episodic illness and chronic conditions (4).

British Columbia Primary Health Care is defined as the point at which a person enters the health care system and receives the health care services that meet most of their everyday needs (5).

Manitoba Primary Health Care is defined as first level contact with the health system where services are mobilized to promote health, prevent illnesses, care for common illnesses, and manage ongoing health problems. It includes all human services that play a part in addressing the interrelated factors that affect health (6).

Nova Scotia Primary Health Care Renewal focuses on improvements in population health and allows citizens to select a primary health care provider and access a range of primary health care services (7).

Ontario Primary Care Reform has created family health networks to deliver primary care. Groups of physicians, supplemented with a nurse-staffed telephone service 24 hours a day, emphasize comprehensive care while promoting a stronger doctor-patient relationship (8).

Prince Edward Island focuses on primary health services described as those services that people access first and most often, such as family physicians, public health nursing, screening programs, addiction services, and community mental health services (9).

Despite the different terminology and varying degrees of scope in provincial plans, there are a number of common elements consistently referenced in the policy documents. They are:

- *Team approach to service delivery:* this is loosely defined given that some provinces begin with the family physician and build other providers around him or her whereas other provinces start with a nurse or nurse practitioner and use medical resources at the next stage of contact.

- *Roster of patients:* there is a general desire to get patients registered with a specific group practice or team of providers. There appears to be varying degrees of formality about this aspect of reform with some provinces talking about "sign-up" periods and others not limiting patient movement among different providers in any way.
- *Twenty-four hour access seven days a week:* this commitment appears to be largely after-hours access to a nurse by telephone.
- *Mixed funding formulas for services and programs:* there is fairly mild experimentation being proposed for new funding models such as capitation, salary, and combinations of such in conjunction with fee-for-service payments. A number of provinces are proposing to move to a population-based funding model linked to specific demographic and health characteristics of enrolled populations.
- *Increased emphasis on health promotion and prevention:* all the provinces' policy materials emphasize a focus on health promotion and prevention.

If we take these common elements as a loose Canadian "model," we can examine the barriers and facilitators to implementation.

ANALYTIC FRAMEWORK

Three variables are proposed for the barriers and facilitators analysis:

- the legacy of Canadian health policy culture,
- the structure and design of Canadian health care,
- the supports required for policy implementation.

Canadian Health Policy Culture

The Canadian health policy culture is not an environment in which rapid change is easily achieved. Various policy legacies exist which affect the ability of leaders to lead change in positive and negative ways.

Barriers. Ten years ago health reform efforts highlighted the need for better integration, coordination, and multidisciplinary care for primary care services. The solution offered by experts was to reform physician payment mechanisms with a shift toward capitation and other alternative payment schemes (10–13). The focus on physician payment was not surprising as medical services are publicly funded and are therefore the logical entry point for governments to lever change.

The language has not changed dramatically over the decade — integration, coordination, and multidisciplinary care are still the policy descriptors for reform. And not surprisingly, the legacy of a focus on physician payment remains. Current efforts of primary care reform are organized around services provided by physicians, albeit in conjunction with others, and funding flows to the physician or group of physicians, not to patients or other health professionals.

Embedded within the history of physician payment in Canada is another legacy — that of paying physicians on a fee-for-service basis. Physicians entered Canadian medicare on the basis of existing fee schedules — a price for each service delivered. Although some experimentation has occurred over time, and physicians are indicating an increasing willingness to consider alternative forms of payment (14), fee-for-service is still the primary way in which primary care services are funded. Alternate payments only account for 11 percent of total clinical earnings in Canada (15). Fee-for service payment is predicated on single services delivered by one professional at a time. It does not facilitate care delivered holistically or delivered by teams of professionals and it does not compensate for time spent for administrative, managerial, educational or communication tasks.

Most expert reviews and some of the evaluations from the Health Transition Fund have identified the need to move away from fee-for-service payment in varying degrees (4,16). Yet movement away from fee-for-service payment is not endorsed by provincial medical associations — the bargaining agents for Canadian physicians. Provincial governments have not, to date, been prepared to implement new funding models over the objections of the medical profession. And, because negotiations are bipartite between governments and medical associations, there is no opportunity for the influence and views of other health professions to be considered as part of allocation decisions.

A third legacy of the culture of Canadian health policy is the use of pilot projects. Rather than move to full implementation, provincial governments often attempt policy reforms of new initiatives through pilot projects. This often gives an impression that a final decision on a policy direction hasn't been made, permits time for opposition to build, and leaves open the possibility of policy reversal when new ministers or governments take office. Primary care reform in Canada is being introduced largely through pilot or demonstration projects.

Facilitators. While Canadian health policy culture has created some legacy problems for primary care reform, it also contains several positive legacies that could contribute to successful implementation.

Canadians are open to new models of care and service delivery and have been for some time. They are aware that a range of providers would benefit their health and are willing to consider their first point of contact with a primary health care system to be with someone other than a physician (17,18). And while Canadians clearly want to maintain a close connection to a personal family physician, they also use a wide variety of other professionals and pay for their services directly (19).

Canadians have also expressed a strong interest in health promotion and prevention activities (20) which supports the thrust of current provincial efforts.

Structure and Design

The structure and design of Canadian health care creates some difficulties for implementing new models as well as opportunities.

Barriers. Although primary care design is being touted as an integrated reform, a closer look at actual implementation plans indicates that this is not the case; indeed, it could not be the case under current legislative arrangements. Neither funding models or provincial health professions regulatory frameworks are structurally supportive of primary care reform.

Federal funding covers only portions of the comprehensive services being envisioned for primary care. Some services are funded under the *Canada Health Act* (e.g., physician services), some are funded through specific federal-provincial programmatic arrangements (e.g., pharmacare), and some are covered only by individual provinces (e.g., alternative health professionals). As well, funding at the provincial level is not always in one pot. For example, Ontario Family Health Networks must work through a different part of the Ministry of Health with a different funding stream to access nurse practitioner funding. Because funding is tied to providers rather than patients, it is not integrated. Attempting to implement new delivery models on the existing hodge-podge of funding arrangements cannot support integration and team-based care.

On the regulatory side, health professions legislation is based on distinct professions each with educational requirements, practice standards, and regulatory colleges. There is no common approach even in areas of overlapping scopes of practice. Professional liability schemes are focused on individuals rather than teams and are legally based on professional autonomy rather than shared accountability. As well, increased specialization and calls for continually higher levels of educational certification as entry qualifications to practice would appear to be decreasing rather than increasing integration and team-based care.

Facilitators. One of the most positive facilitators for implementing primary care is the role played by the Primary Health Care Transition Fund. Initial evaluation reports are now available and make clear that much was learned about implementation at the local level from the providers' and patients' perspectives. Although many felt more time was required to undertake actual implementation, they were positive about new models of delivery (4,16). This evidence provides a good basis for enlarging the scope of activity and the number of participants across the country.

Second, provincial governments have wisely chosen to offer a number of delivery models allowing providers to choose the model they feel best suits their individual circumstances and allowing patients to change care providers if they wish. Although this likely lengthens the time required for implementation, it leaves providers feeling more in control of their practice arrangements and that the decision to change was theirs. It also makes it more likely that patients will enrol.

Required Supports for Policy Implementation

Change-management literature tells us that certain supports are required to implement change. Things such as personnel and skills, appropriate resources, and information technology are needed to support a desired policy change.

Barriers. Health human-resources planning has become an urgent policy issue for the Canadian health care system in the last five years. In particular, national strategies for physician and nursing personnel have been recommended. This is difficult to do in the absence of a clear vision for primary care and some consistency across provincial jurisdictions. Without a stronger link between national health human-resource planning and local primary care delivery, implementation of primary care may be less than optimal. For example, a greater use of nurse practitioners is clearly envisioned but to date increased training slots and new funding models have not materialized.

Information technology has been recognized as a necessary support to clinical integration and improved health outcomes and governments are investing in varying degrees. However, initial projects indicate the costs of real-time information technology are more than anticipated (4,16). This may deter some governments from province-wide implementation or slow down the time frame.

Another potential barrier is expressed concerns about the privacy of the health information that will be shared across practitioners or networks in the new delivery models. Although there is no evidence that the information will be any less secure than in current primary care settings, citizens do occasionally raise the issue and privacy legislation specific to health information is being introduced or implemented in a number of provinces. Primary care reform efforts will need to ensure compliance with new legislative requirements and take into account citizens' sensitivities.

Facilitators. There are a number of supports in place for primary care reform that will likely facilitate implementation. New funding is being made available at the federal and provincial levels. Health information systems are being put in place to support changed delivery. Initial reports from early adopters of the new models are positive both from the provider and the patient perspective. And, some provinces have new health professions legislation that provides a more flexible regulatory scheme to take advantage of the full scope of practice of non-physician personnel.

WHY HAS IMPLEMENTATION BEEN SLOW?

Although we often use the term health care system, Canadians don't really have a system. Each province and territory has its own particular set of programs, models, funding rules, and so on. Primary care is no different. Whatever the design for primary care in any particular jurisdiction, it is still viewed as a program on its own. It is still not connected to other parts of the health care system such as mental health services, long-term care facilities, or home-care programs.

Until a systems approach is taken that integrates the constitute elements of health care, primary care reform will likely be slow. Change is being attempted on a number of levels with somewhat competing demands for attention, resources, and public support. It is difficult to see where the priority lies at present. This is combined with four-year electoral cycles that negate political will to change the closer the election call becomes. Therefore, there are actually very short windows of opportunity to undertake reform, particularly when those affected are not entirely supportive of all aspects of the change.

Given these conditions, it is not surprising that primary care implementation has been slow and arduous.

CONCLUSIONS — IS IT IMPOSSIBLE?

Despite the difficult policy environment, a number of factors have aligned which make the likelihood of success stronger as we begin 2004 than it has been historically. These factors include:

- there is an evidence-base for some of the elements of the reform packages;
- citizens are interested in comprehensive and accessible primary care services;
- a growing number of health professionals are expressing interest in new models of care and are participating in projects;
- the required supports are coming on-line, albeit slowly.

Perhaps the question now is not why has implementation been slow, but rather how patient are we prepared to be?

REFERENCES

1   Hutchsion B, Abelson J, Lavis J. Primary care in Canada: so much innovation, so little change. Health Affairs 2001; 20(3):116–131.

2   Lamarche PA, Beaulieu MD, Pineault R, Contandriopoulos AP, Denis JL, Haggerty J. Choices for change: The path for restructuring primary healthcare services in Canada. Final report. Ottawa: Canadian Health Services Research Foundation; 2003. Available at http:www.chsrf.ca/search_e.php

3   Marriott J, Mable AL. Opportunities and potential. A review of international literature on primary health care reform and models. Ottawa: Health Canada; August 2000.

4   Alberta Health and Wellness. Advancing primary health care in Alberta, sharing the learning: primary health care as a model: lessons learned. Edmonton: Alberta Health and Wellness; 2001.

5   BC Health Planning. Primary health care renewal in BC. Available at http://www.healthservices.gov.bc.ca/phc/phc_materials.htm/#primer

6   Manitoba Health. Primary health care reform in Manitoba. Available at http://www.gov.mb.ca/health/primaryhealth.html

7   Nova Scotia. Department of Health. Primary health care renewal. Available at http://www.gov.ns.ca/health/phcrenewal/vision/htm

8   Ontario. Ministry of Health and Long-Term Care. Primary care reform in Ontario. http://www.health.gov.on.ca/english/public/updates.archives/hu_03/docnurse/ pricare_fs.html

9   Prince Edward Island. Department of Health and Social Services. Pathways to wellness and sustainability — strategic plan for PEI health and social services system 2001-2005. Available at http://www.gov.pe.ca/publications/

10   Ontario Health Review Panel. Toward a shared direction for health in Ontario. Toronto; the Panel; 1987.

11   British Columbia Royal Commission on Health Care and Costs. Closer to home. Victoria: Government of British Columbia; 1991.

12   Premier's Commission on Future Health Care for Albertans. The rainbow report: our vision for health. Edmonton: the Commission; 1989.

13   Nova Scotia. Department of Health and Fitness. Minister's Implementation Committee. Health strategy for the nineties: managing better health. Halifax; the Department; 1990.

14   Canadian Medical Association. Results of the CMA's 2003 Physician Resource Questionnaire. Available at http://www.cmaj.ca/cgi/data/169/7/701/DC1/23

15   Canadian Institute for Health Information. Health care in Canada 2003. Ottawa: CIHI; 2003.

16   Knock M. Primary care demonstration project. Final report to the Health Transition Fund. Ottawa: BC Primary Care Reform Project; 31 March 2001.

17   Maxwell J, Jackson K, Legowski B, Rosell S, Yankelovich D. Report on citizens' dialogue on the future of health care in Canada. Saskatoon: Commission on the Future of Health Care in Canada; 2002.

18   Pollara. Health care in Canada survey 2002. Available at http://www.polara.ca/New/Library/SURVEYS/Healthcare2002.pdf

19   Pollara. Public input on the future of health care in Canada. Saskatoon: Commission on the Future of Health Care in Canada; 2002.

20   Fooks C and Maslove L. Understanding public views on concepts of population health and health determinants. Submitted to Canadian Population Health Initiative (CPHI). September 2003.

Organizing Primary Care Reform

Getting Doctors to Work Together and with Others

Marie-Dominique Beaulieu

In order to help translate ideas into concrete actions, some of us were asked to propose some specific ways to implement the key components of primary care reform, given our understanding of the current barriers to and facilitators of a successful process of change in this area.

The success of primary care reform depends on several interrelated components: (i) funding primary care and the need to find more appropriate ways to remunerate professionals, namely physicians; (ii) strengthening the bonds between users and primary care settings and providers; (iii) and developing effective information technology (IT) to support integration of care. Getting doctors to work in groups and developing interdisciplinary work amongst primary care professionals have been identified as key components as well (1–3). In this chapter I will focus on group practice and interdisciplinary work in primary care, and I will allude to some of the other important components of primary care reform as they relate to these two issues.

Many frameworks for successful change in organizations have been proposed. I will use the one proposed by Contandriopoulos et al. (4). According to this framework, the change process is anchored in three components:

- The "project" to be implemented: is it clearly defined, consensual, perceived as a solution to the problem? How wide is the gap between the current reality and the desired model?

- The "competencies and leadership" needed to implement the change: do the actors involved in making the change possess the required skills? Is there sufficient leadership at the different levels of decision making concerned by the change to solve problems as they occur?
- Are the necessary "resources" available, be they financial, human or technological?

Having this framework in mind, the chapter is organized around the following questions:

- What do we mean by group practice and interdisciplinary teamwork; in other words, what is the project we are working on?
- What are the conditions of success? What barriers have been encountered? What competencies, leadership and resources are needed?
- Issues and challenges: what are the next steps that will move change forward?

GETTING DOCTORS TO WORK TOGETHER: GROUP PRACTICE AND NETWORKS

What Is the Project? Where Do We Stand?

"Without a sense of shared purpose, a group is simply a complicated and unmanageable collection of doctors who have been accustomed to achieving success of their own" (5). To organize primary care, you need organizations to work with. It is not a small challenge when a major element of the relevant work force, family physicians, are not organized as such. Hence, the importance attributed to group practice (5). Group practice is seen as an essential stepping stone to solving problems with access to primary care, continuity of care, integrating quality of care systems in primary care settings, and creating accountability processes between the parts of the health care system responsible for primary care and primary care physicians (1,2).

However, the concept of group practice is much more than the mere association in the same premises of a collection of physicians. To reach its full potential, group practice must have the following characteristics: shared vision, shared clientele, shared tasks and activities, shared expenses, shared revenues, and quality assurance (5). Where do we stand in Canada on these issues? According to the last report by the Canadian Institute of Health Information (CIHI) (6) 70 percent of family physicians in Canada work in some form of group practice. If, at first glance, this appears a good mark, a closer look at the data is disturbing. It is actually in cities, where the problems with continuity and coordination of care are thought to be more acute, that we find a higher proportion of family physicians working solo (up to 46 percent). Moreover, the data does not allow for a good understanding of the conditions of group practice for the 70 percent who describe themselves as working in groups, but it is believed that group practices with the desired characteristics are not the norm.

Another concept which has been put forward to support primary care reform is "practice networks." Although both concepts are not mutually exclusive — indeed, group practices may join in a given area to form a network — they are different. Recognizing the reluctance of some family physicians to work in groups, the College of Family Physicians of Canada (CFPC) has proposed in its " Prescription for Renewal" (3) the concept of Family Practice Networks (FPNs). Networks are composed of physicians working in "actual" or "virtual" groups, linked through IT to facilitate transfer of information. They share some clinical responsibilities, namely 24/7 coverage, and could work together to provide some clinical services in order to deliver, as a network, the full "basket" of primary care services. They are also accountable to some form of regional or local health authority. Interestingly enough, no model proposes formal registration of clients as an inherent characteristic.

Examples of both kinds of "groupings" of family physicians presently exist in Canada. The "Groupes de médecine familiale" (or Family Medicine Groups) in Quebec, and the Ontario Family Health Network relate to the philosophy of group practice, while the Ontario Family Health Groups and the Alberta Primary Care Initiative, place more emphasis on the FPN model. To date, the Ontario Family Health Groups Networks are the only initiatives that have registration of patients as an inherent characteristic of the model.

Conditions of Success and Barriers: Competencies, Resources and Leadership

There are many incentives for physicians to work in groups or networks, most of them being professional incentives rather than financial ones. Improvement in quality of life, improvement in the quality of care offered to patients, as well as access to information technologies have been reported and observed as the most powerful incentives (7).

Interestingly enough, the obstacles to group practice have not been studied in great depth. A study conducted in Belgium and France, two countries trying to organize their general practitioners, who have a strong tradition of independent practice, identified several obstacles. The physicians surveyed believed the necessity of sharing the same vision of care, sharing patients and income as well as collaborating on 24/7 coverage — thus restricting their autonomy in time planning — are important obstacles to group practice (8). Fear of government intrusion is also perceived as a major obstacle, strong enough to undermine the professional incentives of group practice. This last obstacle has also been expressed by some family physicians in Canada, in addition to other constraints inherent in the process of getting organized (mainly the time and effort required in order to "get your act together") (9).

Evaluations of the many initiatives undertaken in Canada during the first wave of the Health Transition Fund highlight some of the conditions necessary for group practice and networks to succeed (10,11). They are summarized in Table 1.

TABLE 1

CONDITIONS NECESSARY FOR SUCCESSFUL GROUP PRACTICE AND NETWORKS

- Strong leadership from local family physicians, with a "champion" to lead the work
- A primary care structure at the regional level that can engage the medical leadership and work with it
- A regional authority committed to primary care, which:
  - maintains focus on the vision within the organization, particularly to arbitrate competing priorities with other sectors;
  - manages the change process and the local dynamics through its managerial resources;
  - creates professional incentives (breaks isolation, supports continuing education, etc);
  - compensates financial losses (particularly time devoted to meetings).

Issues and Challenges for Group Practice and Networks

Going back to the framework for change proposed in the introduction, we can say that, even if there are some variations in the models of group practice proposed, there is a relative professional consensus on the "projects" of group practice and networks. It can also be argued that getting doctors to work together bears on competencies that are known to the medical profession. Moving forward will be more a question of leadership, resources, and managerial competencies. Some questions remain, which will have to be addressed while following up on the projects presently under way in Canada. For instance, what will be the outcomes of the different models implemented in terms of accessibility and continuity? In other words, will the models with fewer constraints and incentives accomplish comparable results? Is there some compromise with respect to patient registration? Could "accreditation of practices" according to some processes and targeted outcomes, a model undertaken in Australia (12) but not considered in Canada, have comparable results? How will we create a culture of quality assurance in primary care settings? To date, there is no systematic move in Canada in this direction. Can we achieve the full potential of group practice without quality assurance systems? Some think not (5,7).

GETTING DOCTORS WORKING WITH OTHERS: INTERDISCIPLINARY PRIMARY CARE TEAMS

What Is the Project? Where Do We Stand?

"... family physicians, nurse practitioners, nurses, midwives and other health care professionals would work in interdisciplinary, integrated teams" (3). This quotation could have been taken from the report of the Commission on the Future of Health Care in Canada (1), or any other report produced to date, with the exception of the Clair Report (2) which is more indicative of what constitutes the "core" primary care team: six to ten family physicians working with two "clinical" nurses (the profession of nurse practitioner is not recognized in Quebec). The point is, while we are relatively clear on what a "group practice" is, the "interdisciplinary team" approach is a fuzzier concept and does not mean the same thing to all. According to CIHI's latest report (6), only 7 percent of family physicians practising within groups report that they work with nurse practitioners, and 27 percent with other health professionals. The proportions are lower for physicians working in solo practices and in walk-in clinics. It is in Quebec, with the Centres locaux de services communautaires (CLSCs), that experience with multidisciplinary work is most common. However, some studies have revealed important problems of collaboration within this context (13,14). Still, the Canadian population is favourable to the idea of teamwork: in a survey conducted for the Romanow Commission, 54 percent of those surveyed responded that they would be ready to consult a nurse who works with a family physician and 49 percent think that primary care teams would improve health (6).

Some argue that getting doctors to work within teams is not a problem per se, because physicians are used to working with other health professionals.

After all, physicians have experienced "teamwork" during their training, working daily on hospital wards and clinics with other health professionals. It would be interesting to poll physicians about their perception of teamwork, based on their experiences. We could be surprised to find that it can differ substantially from one individual to another.

Experiences with multidisciplinary or interdisciplinary teams can be described from the perspective of the clientele they intend to reach, or the setting in which they take place, or a mixture of both. In my view, the models that emerge from these experiences can fit within different categories. We have what we can call a "vulnerable clientele model," for instance, the frail elderly with various handicaps or palliative care patients. Often developed within the hospital setting, which lends itself more to formal and informal teamwork, this model has been extended and implemented with some success in ambulatory-care settings (15). This model could be seen as the "heavy artillery" model. It is a model where much of the work on interdisciplinary practices — its prerequisites, its drawbacks and difficulties — has been done (16). It would be tempting, but probably misleading, to lean on these experiences to develop a vision of what a primary care team may represent. The mere thought of such a complex model might frighten many family physicians.

Another model could be described as the "disease management" model, a model developed in specialty ambulatory care settings. The focus is on treatment of a specific disease, it bears on the central role of a case manager, usually a nurse, working in close relationship with specialists and other professionals. Linkage with family physicians is not the hallmark of those models (17). Considering the importance of co-morbidity in most patients with chronic conditions, some have identified a risk of fragmentation if such a model was to be the "reference" model for primary care (17).

Finally, we have what can be described as the "intensive-care-unit/emergency-room" model. It is the model which physicians have most experience with, and probably the one they refer to (and like) most when they think of primary care teams. While the utility of this model is certain, it relies on what could be called a "directive" model of teamwork rather than a collaborative one. It is not the model of reference for most health care professionals who want to engage in interdisciplinary work, and probably not the most appropriate in terms of what would constitute an effective new may of "re-engineering" primary care teams (18–20).

Some interesting experiences are underway in Canada. There is the work of Way and Jones who have tried to develop collaborative practices between family physicians and nurse practitioners in Ontario. Although promising, the experience has fallen short of producing strong collaborative practices (21).

We have to turn to the United Kingdom to find illustrations of the most interesting experiences of primary care teams. Many models actually exist there, with a variety of professionals and nurses, and they are evolving in the wake of the new Primary Care Trusts initiatives. The intent of the present discussion is not to suggest that one model of primary care team and collaboration will fit all settings. However, it is clear that there is still considerable work to be done in refining the concept if we want to move from a "motherhood and apple pie" statement to a clear "blueprint."

Conditions of Success and Barriers: Competencies, Resources and Leadership

This section will address two topics: the conditions of fruitful interdisciplinary work and obstacles overcome and the solutions found by those engaged in this endeavour in the context of primary care reform in Canada.

First, what do we know of the conditions of effective interdisciplinary work in primary care? Research on primary care teams is scant. In a systematic review of 136 studies on interdisciplinary teams, Schofield and Amodeo (16) concluded that few studies have tried to link the characteristics of teams — number of professionals, remuneration methods, and processes of collaboration — with outcomes. Most studies relied on ill-defined frameworks of interdisciplinary work and used weak designs. None was conducted in primary care. We can find guidance in the work conducted by Poulton and West on the effectiveness of teamwork (22,23) which has been recently applied by Campbell et al. in the context of general practice in the United Kingdom (24). The authors were able to link characteristics of positive "team climate" to effectiveness of health outcomes for the management of patients with asthma. The characteristics were participation, clear and shared objectives, support for innovation, and a focus on quality of care.

However, experiences with teamwork have taken place in specific health care systems and a good understanding of the conditions of successful interdisciplinary work has to take into account a more systemic view. The work by Lamarche and colleagues, who have taken a configurational approach to the study of primary care organizations, reveals that if multidisciplinary work is one of the characteristics of primary care models that attain the best configuration of outcomes, it is not the only one (25). Key components are also related to the way primary care is funded, the presence of strong incentives to promote "vertical integration" of care, remuneration of physicians that does not depend only on fee-for-service, and a strong emphasis on information and diagnostic technologies. In summary, there is no magic bullet for primary care teams. Great attention should be given to the development of a clear and shared vision of teamwork, to the processes teams will put in place, and the general organizational context in which they develop.

What are the obstacles met by those who have engaged in such initiatives in the scope of primary care reform in Canada? Again, lessons can be drawn from the synthesis of the Health Transition Fund initiatives (10,11) as well as from the proceedings of a conference on primary care teams conducted in 2002 in Montreal (9). These obstacles are summarized in Table 2. On the other hand, the conditions of fruitful collaboration can be identified (9,18,19) (Table 3). It requires leadership at all levels and competencies both in the area of collaborative practice and in the area of effective change management.

TABLE 2

OBSTACLES TO THE DEVELOPMENT OF INTERDISCIPLINARY TEAMWORK IN THE CONTEXT OF PRIMARY CARE REFORM

- Contradictory messages on goals and conflicting timetables from various decision-making levels; often takes the form of the political level asking for rapid results when the practitioners need more time to develop the models at the local level.
- Resistance in the field which built on
  - distrust and opposition to the models proposed (which actually were often combining issues related to group practice in addition to issues related to interdisciplinary work);
  - differences in culture and practice styles;
  - and, must one say, ignorance of each others' competencies.
- Financial, legal, and regulatory frameworks incongruent with the objectives.
- Lack of support in the management of change.

TABLE 3

CONDITIONS FOR FRUITFUL COLLABORATION

- an explicit relationship of trust
- a focus on what is at stake: good patient care
- a clear vision of "who does what"
- mechanisms to support teamwork
- interdisciplinary training

Issues and Challenges for Interdisciplinary Teams in Primary Care

It is an understatement to say that the plate is full for those who want to develop primary care teams. Work has to be done on all aspects of the change framework. Work must be done on refining the project in order to facilitate a common understanding of the vision and a clear definition of roles. This occurs in a period when family physicians are looking for new directions and may feel threatened by proposals that cut them off from what they perceive as an essential aspect of their work: ongoing care and counselling based on a strong doctor-patient relationship. The professional uneasiness of family physicians with some of the proposals put forward should not be underestimated, for fear is a major barrier to change. In refining the "project" of primary care teams, two challenges will have to be met:

- The integration of the "chronic care model" which has been developed from disease management in a broader primary care model that encompasses both dealing with the follow-up of patients with co-morbidity and the daily management of common conditions and new problems (17).
- A constant preoccupation with making teamwork "visible" to patients, to prevent the feeling of "fragmentation" reported by some patients who receive their care from more structured primary care organizations (26).

Finally, there is a major need for competency development. In that endeavour, professional associations, colleges, and universities are key players. Leadership will have to be strong at all levels, for professionals willing to engage in these primary care initiatives will not have the leverage to counter alone important obstacles related to regulations and financial compensation.

REFERENCES

1   Commission on the Future of Health Care in Canada. RJ Romanow, Commissioner. Building on values: the future of health care in Canada – final report. Ottawa: the Commission; 2002.
2   Quebec. Study Commission on Health and Social Services. Emerging solutions: report and recommendations. Quebec: the Commission; 2000.
3   College of Family Physicians of Canada. Primary care and family medicine in Canada: a prescription for renewal. Mississauga: College of Family Physicians of Canada; 2000.
4   Contandriopoulos AP, Champagne F, Denis JL, Avargues MC. L'évaluation dans le domaine de la santé: concepts et méthodes. Revue d'épidémiologie et de santé publique 2000;48:517–539.
5   Cincotta JA. Developing "group thinking" in a multispeciality group. Family Practice Management 1999;6:45–49.

6   Canadian Institute for Health Information. Health care in Canada. Ottawa: CIHI; 2003.

7   Hawks AN. A case study in developing a successful medical group. American Academy of Family Physicians 1999;6:42–45.

8   Feron JM, Cerexhe F, Pestiaux D, Roland M, Giet D, Montrieux C, et al. GP's working in solo practice: obstacles and motivations for working in a group? A qualitative study. Family Practice 2003;20:167–172.

9   Beaulieu MD, Goudreau J, Denis JL, Millette B, D'Amour D, Lebeau R. The team in primary care: a new vision, new ways to work. Record of Proceedings of the Colloquium sponsored by the Doctor Sadok Besrour Chair in Family Medicine. Montreal; 2003.

10   Mable AL, Marriott J. The Health Transition Fund. Primary health care. Ottawa: Health Canada Health Transition Fund; 2002.

11   Desbiens F, Dagenais C, Joubert P. De l'innovation au changement: Les leçons tirées des projets québécois financés par le Fonds pour l'adaptation des services de santé (FASS). Montréal: Ministère de la Santé et des Services sociaux; 2001.

12   Modra C, Whaites L, Kalycy E. Ten years on — results of the 2001-2002 Annual Survey of Divisions of General Practice. Adelaide: Department of General Practice, Flinders University, and Commonwealth Department of Health and Ageing; 2003.

13   D'Amour D. Structuration de la collaboration interprofessionnelle dans les services de santé de première ligne au Québec. Thèse pour le doctorat en Santé publique. Montréal: GRIS; 1997.

14   Sicotte C, D'Amour D, Moreau MP. Interdisciplinary collaboration within Quebec community health care centres. Social Science and Medicine 2002;55:991–1003.

15   Leatt P. Integrated service delivery. Synthesis Series. Ottawa: Health Canada Health Transition Fund; 2002.

16   Schofield RF, Amodeo M. Interdisciplinary teams in health care and human settings: are they effective? Health and Social Work 1999;24:210–219.

17   Rothman AA, Wagner EH. Chronic illness management: what is the role of primary care? Annals of Internal Medicine 2003;138:256–261.

18   MacIntosh J, McCormack D. Partnerships identified within primary health care literature. International Journal of Nursing Studies 2001;38:547–555.

19   Way D, Jones L, Busing N. Implementation strategies: collaboration in primary care — family doctors and nurse practitioners delivering shared care. Toronto: Ontario College of Family Physicians; 2000.

20   Richards A, Carley J, Jenkins-Clarke S, Richards DA. Skill mix between nurses and doctors working in primary care — delegating or allocation: a review of the literature. International Journal of Nursing Studies 2000;37:185–197.

21   Way D, Jones L, Baskerville B, Busing N. Primary health care services provided by nurse practitioners and family physicians in shared practice. Canadian Medical Association Journal 2001;165:1210–1214.

22   Poulton BC, West MA. Primary health care team effectiveness: developing a constituency approach. Health & Social Care in the Community 1993;2:77–84.

23   Poulton BC, West MA. The determinants of effectiveness in primary health care teams. Journal of Interprofessional Care 1999;13:7–18.

24   Campbell SM, Hann J, Hacker J, Burns BJ, Olivier D, Thapar A, et al. Identifying predictors of high quality care in English general practice: observational study. British Medical Journal 2001;323:784–787.

25   Lamarche P, Beaulieu M-D, Pineault R , Contandriopoulos A-P, Denis J-L, Haggerty J. Choices for change: the path for restructuring primary healthcare services in Canada. Ottawa: Canadian Health Services Research Foundation: 2003. Available at http:// www.chsrf.ca/search_e.php

26   Safran DG. Defining the future of primary care: what can we learn from patients? Annals of Internal Medicine 2003;138:248–255.

Summing Up

Primary Health Care Reform in Contemporary Health Care Systems

Barbara Starfield

From an international viewpoint, primary health care has been on the agenda for twenty-five years. In 1978, the World Health Organization held a conference in Alma Ata (then the Soviet Union) that affirmed the importance of primary care as the basis of health systems. Recognizing "the existing gross inequalities in health" and that "the promotion and protection of health is essential to sustained economic and social development," the Declaration of Alma Ata stated that "All governments should formulate national policies, strategies, and plans of action to launch and sustain primary health care as part of a comprehensive national system and in coordination with other sectors" (1).

The Alma Ata definition was very broad in its conceptualization of primary health care, including activities generally considered to be part of public health, e.g., clean water and appropriate sewage management, as well as personal health services. Thus, primary health care has two component parts: activities targeted to populations and activities targeted to individuals within populations. Both categories focus on populations; they differ only in the extent to which interventions themselves are directed at the population (or subpopulations) as a whole, or at individuals within the population (2). For example, legislation to mandate folic acid supplementation in flour, or regulations to reduce air pollutants, do not require any interaction with or of individuals to improve health. In contrast, mandatory immunizations require individual actions, even though they are directed at populations. Implementation of clinical guidelines is similarly focused on individuals, albeit within particular subpopulations.

The term primary care, as distinguished from primary health care, is generally reserved for the clinical activity that primarily focuses on individuals. The distinction between the two is, however, narrowing over time as primary care facilities and programs increasingly assume responsibility for maintaining and improving the health of defined populations.

Unfortunately for the Alma Ata declaration, it came at the wrong time. The era of market reform, lasting from the beginning of the 1980s through the 1990s, shifted attention to hospitals, specialization, and the increased used of technology and pharmaceuticals. The recommendations of the World Health Organization were disregarded by many countries.

The failures of the market-oriented reforms to constrain rapidly increasing costs of care, as well as an aging population, high prevalence of chronic diseases, the emergence of new and highly infectious acute diseases with chronic sequelae, recognition of the high frequency of co-morbidity, and increasing inequity in health both within and across countries have been responsible for a revival of interest in primary health care.

In May of 2003, the World Health Assembly directed the World Health Organization to request member states to "ensure the development of primary health care is adequately resourced in order to contribute to the reduction in health inequalities; and to strengthen human resource capability for primary health care to tackle the rising burdens of health conditions." WHO was instructed to convene a meeting with input from all stakeholders to examine the lessons of the past 25 years, review definitions and strategies, and identify future strategic directions for primary health care." The director-general was requested to report on progress to the Fifty-seventh World Health Assembly, through the executive board, at its thirteenth session in May 2004 (3).

As a result, the regional offices of WHO held meetings to discuss the role of primary health care within health systems. In October of 2003, a conference was held in Madrid, Spain, to consider the individual regional efforts and develop an international proposal for consideration by the executive board of WHO and subsequently by the 2004 World Health Assembly. While the exact shape of the resulting decisions and actions cannot be predicted at the time of this writing, there is little doubt of the widespread interest in primary care in most countries of the world.

There is ample reason to focus on primary care. A wealth of evidence, both within and across countries, points to better effectiveness at lower costs when primary care is adequate. Three studies (one of which replicated a prior study) were large international comparisons across industrialized nations. The first of these reported on ten Organisation for Economic and Cultural Development (OECD) countries, which were ranked on nine characteristics related to primary care, five of which concerned characteristics of the health system conducive to primary care practice and six of which concerned characteristics of primary care practice in the country (4). In this study, costs were notably lower in countries that scored high on primary care characteristics. These countries had better health levels on average, as assessed by 15 measures of mortality and morbidity. The repeat study, approximately five years later (mid-1990s) added six additional system characteristics and three additional countries. It confirmed the inverse association between primary care strength and costs of care and, additionally, demonstrated the benefits of primary care, which were most notable for indicators in infancy and childhood. In contrast with the widespread perception of the US health system as producing the best health in the world for its population, these studies showed the United States to rank last or near last on all indicators except those late in life (life expectancy at ages 65, 80, and 85). Ranking of the countries on other characteristics often associated with health levels (e.g., smoking rates, degree of income inequality) failed to find them a competing explanation for the findings across the countries (5).

A more recent and technically sophisticated study examined the relationship between the strength of focus on primary care (using scores similar to those used in the previous studies) and health status, after controlling for gross domestic product, percent elderly, physicians per capita, average income (in purchasing power parities), and alcohol and tobacco use. A significant relationship with primary care score was found for all cause mortality; life expectancy; infant mortality; potential years of life lost (PYLL) for all causes, for pneumonia and influenza, for asthma and bronchitis, for cerebrovascular disease, and for heart disease among males, and for all the categories under PYLL in females. The relationship between primary care and the other measures of health in females were in the same direction but did not reach statistical significance. A fixed effects, pooled cross-sectional time series analysis of the same data showed the consistency of these relationships over time, from 1970 through 1998 (6).

In view of the suspicion that the mode of paying physicians might be related to quality of care and perhaps outcomes as well, consideration of this policy-sensitive characteristic has been examined in several studies. In the international comparison reported above, countries rated as poor on primary care all had predominantly fee-for-services arrangements for paying both primary care physicians and specialists. In contrast, all but one of the five countries with the highest primary care scores had various degrees of mixtures between capitation and salary, or capitation and fee-for-service, or salary and fee-for-service arrangements for primary care physicians, even more so in the more recent study than in the earlier one. In all but one of these countries, specialists were paid a salary, being based predominantly in hospital practice. However, all but one of the four countries with intermediate primary care scores and good health statistics after infancy and childhood also paid both primary care physicians and specialists by fee-for-service, suggesting that mode of payment of physician is not responsible for the beneficial effect of primary care (7).

An analysis of information from 21 OECD countries from which data were available and comparable indicated that fee-for-service arrangements in the hospital sector were associated with poor outcomes as reflected in premature mortality in men and women, life expectancy at age 65 in both men and women, perinatal mortality, infant mortality, potential years of life lost from heart disease in men and women, and potential years of life lost from cancer in men and women. There was no clear relationship between mode of payment in the ambulatory sector and health outcomes or costs of care (8).

Results of a controlled trial in a local area in Denmark showed that institution of a fee-for-services system increased the ordering of tests and, hence, greater costs; the impact on outcomes was not assessed (9). Scott and Hall (10) reviewed 18 studies concerning remuneration of primary care physicians. All were consistent in showing an increase in the number of tests and visits; none examined impact on patients' health.

Thus, while fee-for-service mode of payment has not been found to have a direct effect on outcomes of care, it is possible that it has an indirect effect; its cost-increasing effect may result in a situation where fewer resources are available to improve health services, particularly in socially deprived areas.

Other characteristics, however, are more directly related to better health outcomes associated with primary care. In the international comparisons mentioned above, five features – three of them system features amenable to policy change and two practice features – were consistently related to better health outcomes. The system features were attempts to regulate distribution of resources so that areas of need were supplied with resources; financial access to health services assured by a publicly accountable body, e.g., the government; and low or no cost sharing for primary care services. The two practice features were family orientation and comprehensiveness, i.e., the provision, by primary care, of all health care services except those too uncommon for the primary care practitioner to maintain competence in dealing with them. None of the countries with poor primary care and relatively poorer outcomes (especially early in life) had any of these characteristics (5).

This international comparison was also instructive in showing how important health policy is to primary care practice, as there was an almost perfect relationship between ranks of the countries on the system characteristics (which are amenable to health policy decisions) and ranks on the practice characteristics (5). From this finding it is possible to conclude that improving health outcomes requires conducive national health policies.

PRIMARY CARE AND EQUITY IN HEALTH

Until recently, all "models" of influences in health assumed that the pathways to health were the same for individuals as for populations. More recent formulations, motivated by the new international focus on achieving equity in health and health care, recognized the need for models focused on distributions of health in addition to overall (average) levels of health in countries and areas of countries (11,12).

Accumulating evidence on the greater effectiveness of primary care oriented health systems raised questions as to whether the same could be said regarding equity of health and health services. Equity, in the sense used here, means absence of systematic and potentially remediable differences in one or more aspects of health across socially, demographically, or geographically defined population groups (13). Virtually every study has confirmed that primary care oriented health systems increased equity in provision of primary care services. This has been shown in Canada, Sweden, the Netherlands, the United Kingdom (except for preventive services), and the Scandinavian countries as well as in the United States for those 65 years or older (14). However, the same was not the case for use of specialty services, which remains higher for people in less disadvantaged social situations (15–20). It therefore is appropriate to ask whether these differences are associated with better or worse equity in health.

The literature on the subject is sparse. Castro-Leal and colleagues (21) found, from studies in seven African countries, that the highest 20 percent of the population receives well over twice as much financial benefit as the lowest 20 percent from overall government health spending (30 percent vs 12 percent) whereas for primary care spending, the rich-poor benefit is notably lower (23 percent vs 15 percent), leading Gwatkin (22) to conclude that "From an equity perspective, primary care represents a clear step in the right direction."

Additional evidence derives from recent studies of disadvantaged and advantaged subpopulations in industrialized countries. Politzer et al. (23) showed great reductions in low birth weight percentages in people receiving their care in community health centres in the United States. These centres deliver services to populations in underserved geographic areas and are required to maintain standards for high quality of primary care delivery. Most notable was the fact that there were both absolute and relative reductions in low birth weight percentages that were greater in the group with the greatest inequities in the population as a whole (African Americans).

In the US population as a whole, there are large differences in healthy life across racial/ethnic subpopulations, such that low income African Americans and low income Hispanic populations have less healthy life than whole populations. (This measure of health incorporates self-reports of both activity limitation and self-perceived health status. For the former, each person is classified into one of six categories based on age and ability to perform a major activity, other activities, and activities of daily living [ADL]. The combination of the two yielded 30 possible health states which were subjected to psychometric techniques and multi-attribute utility scaling to assign values to each of the 30 states; these ranged from 1, perfect health, to 0.10, for persons limited on ADL and in poor health. If people live one year in excellent health and have no limitation activity, then they have one full year of healthy life. People limited in ADL and in poor health have 10 percent of full function for the year.) In contrast, community health centre (CHC) Hispanic populations have significantly more healthy life than white and African American CHC subpopulations; there are no differences between the latter two groups (24).

A similar study comparing years of healthy life found, as expected, that poor people in the general population had much higher likelihood of fewer years of healthy life; poor CHC patients (who comprise about two-thirds of CHC patients), in contrast, were much closer to non-poor people in years of healthy life (24). A reduction in disparities in health was found when insured were compared with uninsured people; there was no difference in years of healthy life between insured and uninsured people in CHCs, but a large difference in the two groups in the general population with the advantage in the insured people (24).

A series of studies that stratified for degree of income inequality in the United States found lower rates of ill health in those areas with high income inequality that were better endowed with primary care physicians and much worse health in these income inequitable areas if they were poorly endowed with primary care physicians. The measures of health were self-reported health (in 60 representative communities in the US), postneonatal mortality in the 50 US states, and mortality from stroke in the 50 US states (based on data in reference 25).

In the Netherlands, where primary care is well developed, differences in manifestations of ill health between high and low socioeconomic status have been decreasing over time. Mackenbach demonstrated the increase in equity for perinatal mortality between 1946 and 1980, and for infant mortality between 1854 and 1990 (26).

In developing countries, the burden of child mortality, which is most heavily concentrated in disadvantaged populations, can be greatly reduced by interventions known to be effective, all of which are primary care interventions (27,28).

Thus, existing evidence is consistent in showing reductions in health inequities in areas with social inequity that are well endowed with primary care resources. This finding is consistent with the theory that suggests that a strong primary care infrastructure should be more equity-producing. Primary care is less costly than specialized care (4,5,29), thus releasing resources for areas where they are less adequate. Moreover, the important features of primary care practice — accessibility and first contact when needs arise; more person-focused interactions as distinguished from disease-focused interactions; greater comprehensiveness (care for all but uncommon conditions that require referral, and better referral networks); coordination of care when referrals are necessary; family orientation, community orientation, and cultural competence — all are pursuant to an equity agenda (7).

CHALLENGES TO THE ORGANIZATION OF HEALTH SYSTEMS

The benefits of medical care on health, particularly in the most recent half century, are being documented by several investigators (30,31). It is apparent, however, that this effect is limited to appropriate services; it is not across the board. For example, it has been shown that the benefit of specialty services is limited to those aspects of health in the specialist's area of special training (32). Moreover, an increasing supply of specialists above the needed level adds no benefit to health or is actually detrimental (33). For occurrence and/or mortality from colorectal cancer, prostate cancer, and breast cancer, a higher supply of primary care physicians (but not the relevant specialist type) is associated with lower rates (34–36). The reason that increasing specialist rates is adverse is most likely due to inappropriate interventions when there is an excess of resources. Roos (37), for example, showed that outcomes of tonsillectomy and/ or adenoidectomy were better when children were referred to specialists by primary care physicians instead of going directly to specialists.

This evidence on benefit from medical care in general is based on assessment of effect on average health in population. The extent to which it can be assumed to be the case for increasing equity in populations may be debated (14,38–40). At least two reasons may account for this: more disadvantaged patients are less likely to be able to take advantage of new innovations because of poorer access to services, or because they have more co-morbidity (41,42). From a theoretical viewpoint, however, increased benefit of medical care (in general) should improve equity because about three-quarters of the conditions more common among the socially disadvantaged are preventable through early detection of risk (clearly in the primary health care sector); one-quarter are amenable to treatment (some by primary care and some by specialty care) (43). Thus, empirical evidence that primary care is associated with increased equity provides information that the type and appropriateness of services is critical in achieving the desired effect.

CHALLENGES TO PRIMARY AND SPECIALTY CARE IN INCREASING EQUITY IN HEALTH

Three major challenges face both primary care and specialty care in efforts to improve equity in health: achieving high quality primary care; maximizing benefit and minimizing harm from specialty care; and reducing harm from adverse effects of health services interventions.

Achieving high quality primary care. Health policy oriented toward equitable distribution of resources (such that needier areas have more primary care resources), towards guaranteed financial access to primary care services, and low or no co-payments are the basic three characteristics that are amenable to policy changes and authority. The cardinal features of primary care practice (first contact care; person-focused care over time; comprehensiveness of care; coordination of care; community orientation; family-centred; cultural competence) all have demonstrated benefits (7). On the basis of the international comparison reported above, family centredness and comprehensiveness appear to be most critical. The latter of these practice characteristics is highly related to the next challenge for care: developing evidence-based indications for referral to specialists, maintaining the appropriate balance between primary care physicians, and the challenge of coordination of care.

Maximizing benefit and minimizing harm from specialty care. The literature is consistent in showing that specialty care is more appropriate when a primary care physician acts to maximize the justifiability of referral (7, chapter 7;43).

Although referral rates have long been known to be highly variable, very few studies of the phenomenon take into account the possibility that differences in degree of morbidity might account for differences. One relatively recent study remedied that defect by stratifying populations into extent of morbidity burden using a "case-mix" system known as the Johns Hopkins ACG System, which characterizes each individual in the population according to the number of types of illness experienced by each person in a year (44). Data from the United Kingdom were compared with data from five managed care health plans in the US. At each level of morbidity burden, the percentage of patients referred in a year was three times higher in the US managed care plans than in the UK (45). As the analysis stratified the population into groups by morbidity burden, the differences could not be a result of difference in morbidity in the two countries.

Use of specialists in the US increases with increasing morbidity burden (co-morbidity) (46). For individual conditions experienced by patients in a year, the number of visits either to primary care physicians or to specialists does not change with increasing morbidity burden, and the number of visits to primary care physicians exceeds the number to specialists at each level of morbidity. The pattern is the same with regard to visits for co-morbid conditions. However, the number of visits is much higher, and increases steeply with increasing co-morbidity. For populations under the age of 65, the number of visits to primary care physicians exceeds the number of visits to specialists in each co-morbidity group, but the difference is much less than in the case of visits for individual conditions, and lessens with each increase in co-morbidity. That is, the number of visits to specialists for co-morbid conditions more closely approximates (while remaining lower) the number of visits to primary care physicians for co-morbidity, than is the case for visits for individual conditions. For patients over age 65, the pattern for individual conditions is approximately the same, except that the number of visits to specialists slightly exceeds the number of visits to primary care physicians in the highest co-morbidity groups. For co-morbidity, however, the number of visits to specialists exceeds the number of visits to primary care physicians except in the lowest co-morbidity group. At the highest level of co-morbidity, the average number of visits to specialists is about nine per year.

Reid (personal communication 01/03) found that the modal number of specialists seen by the primary care physicians' panels of regular patients was over 100 per year, with the range extending all the way to 400 for a few physicians.

The combination of large numbers of visits to specialists and the large number of specialists with whom primary care physicians have a relationship suggests a major challenge to coordination of care. The presence of co-morbidity adds to this challenge. For example, among patients over age 65, the greater the extent of co-morbidity, the increasingly greater the costs of in-patient care, the number of hospitalizations for conditions that should be preventable by good primary care, and the number of complications occurring in the hospital (47).

The extent of complications, both those due to error and those that are adverse but not known to be related to errors, is associated with considerable mortality, at least in the US.

Reducing adverse effects from medical care. The magnitude of adverse effects of health services interventions leading to death is estimated to be very substantial: 225,000 per year in the United States, or the third leading cause of death (after heart disease and cancer) in that country (48). These estimates derive from studies largely in hospitalized patients. Adverse effects arising in outpatient care are estimated to occur in 4 to 18 percent of consecutive patients (depending on the particular study), at a cost (in the US) of $77 billion per year (equivalent to the total cost of patients with diabetes), and 199,000 deaths (49).

Little, if anything, is known about the extent to which these adverse effects are related to problems in health services delivery (such as failures of coordination), or the extent to which they occur more frequently in socially disadvantaged populations rather than more advantaged ones. Nor is it clear whether they occur preferentially in situations where treatment is inappropriate or unnecessary.

What is abundantly clear, however, is that unnecessary or inappropriate interventions in the US account for 20 to 30 percent of its excessive costs; an additional 20 to 30 percent are administrative costs associated with billing for services (including those that are unnecessary or inappropriate); about 8 percent are attributable to adverse effects, and the remainder to high and rising prices, especially pharmaceuticals, and an aging population (50–53). Excessive supply of specialists in particular geographic areas is associated with higher rates of procedures and testing, to an extent that can only be considered unnecessary as it leads to no better outcomes (15,16)

CONCLUSIONS AND IMPLICATIONS FOR HEALTH POLICY

The following conclusions may be drawn from the above material:

- Primary care is an equity-producing strategy. Countries and areas of countries with poorer primary care resources place socially deprived populations at particular health disadvantage, particularly in the early years of life.
- Specialty use is inequitably distributed in the population (probably everywhere). It is possible that deficits in supply of and use of specialists in areas of relative deprivation compromise the health of socially disadvantaged people through unavailability of needed services.
- Society needs to better understand the appropriate role of specialists and their relationship to primary care providers. The impact of unnecessary or inappropriate use of specialist services is adverse. More informed arrangements for consultation from specialists is warranted.

- Coordination of care is problematic due to the large extent of co-morbidity and the very high use of specialists in people with substantial co-morbidity.
- Adverse effects are most likely a result, at least in part, of coordination problems (as well as individual errors).

There are several implications of these finding for health policy.

- Primary care should be the cornerstone of health systems, as it is especially pursuant to effectiveness, efficiency, and equity. Countries should support the development of World Health Organization policy and activity towards helping nations achieve better primary care infrastructures. In turn, countries should heed WHO policy to better develop their own primary care systems and to encourage the development of primary care systems in other countries.
- Research and development to inform more appropriate use of specialist services should be supported.
- Electronic information systems should be developed with the purpose of improving coordination and reducing adverse effects of interventions.
- Better post-marketing surveillance for adverse effects of new and existing technology, including pharmaceuticals, should be mounted, using electronic information systems and recording and coding of problems (symptoms and signs) in clinical practice.
- The use, in clinical practice and public health, of case-mix systems to routinely characterize the health of people (rather than incidence and prevalence rates of diseases) should be encouraged by health policy. Such systems exist and are ready for use; financial support and incentives for their use and evaluation are warranted.

The world stands on the cusp of a revolution in health services delivery. Unprecedented improvements in health services may increase inequities in health (at the very least) and compromise some aspects of health, at least in some populations. Health policy that encourages equity-producing interventions can be expected to reduce the special disadvantage suffered by socially deprived populations and subpopulations.

REFERENCES

1   World Health Organization. Primary health care. Geneva; 1978. Available at http://www.who.int/hpr/archive/docs/almaata.html Accessed September 4, 2003.

2   Starfield B. Public health and primary care: a framework for proposed linkages. American Journal of Public Health 1996;86(10):1365–1369.

3   World Health Assembly. Resolution Document A56/27. Geneva: World Health Assembly; 2003.

4   Starfield B. Is primary care essential? Lancet 1994;344(8930):1129–1133.

5   Starfield B, Shi L. Policy relevant determinants of health: an international perspective. Health Policy 2002;60(3):201–218.

6   Macinko J, Starfield B, Shi L. The contribution of primary care systems to health outcomes within Organisation for Economic Cooperation and Development (OECD) countries, 1970–1998. Health Services Research 2003;38(3):831–865.

7   Starfield B. Primary care: balancing health needs, services, and technology. New York: Oxford University Press; 1998.

8   Or Z. Exploring the effects of health care on mortality across OECD countries. Labour Market and Social Policy Occasional Papers No. 46. Paris: OECD; 2001.

9   Flierman HA and Groenewegen PP. Introducing fees for services with professional uncertainty. Health Care Finance Review 1992;14(1):107–115.

10   Scott A, Hall J. Evaluating the effects of GP remuneration: problems and prospects. Health Policy 1995;31(3):183–195.

11   Maynard A. Evidence-based medicine: an incomplete method for informing treatment choices. Lancet 1997;349(9045):126–128.

12   Starfield B. Population health: new paradigms and implications for health information systems. In: Friedman DJ, Hunter EL, Parrish RG, editors. Health statistics in the 21st century: implications for health policy and practice. Oxford University Press, 2004. In press.

13   Starfield B. Basic concepts in population health and health care. Journal of Epidemiology and Community Health 2001;55(7):452–445.

14   Dixon A, Legrand J, Henderson J, Murray R, Poteliakhoff E. Is the NHS equitable? a review of the evidence. LSE Health and Social Care Discussion Paper No. 11. London: London School of Economics; 2003.

15   Fisher ES, Wennberg, DE, Stukel TA, Gottlieb DJ, Lucas FL, Pinder EL. The implications of regional variations in medicare spending. Part 1: the content, quality, and accessibility of care. Annals of Internal Medicine 2003;138(4):273–287.

16   Fisher ES, Wennberg DE, Stukel TA, Gottlieb DJ, Lucas FL, Pinder EL. The implications of regional variations in medicare spending. Part 2: health outcomes and satisfaction with care. Annals of Internal Medicine 2003;138(4):288–298.

17   Bongers IM, van der Meer JB, van den Bos J, Mackenbach JP. Socio-economic differences in general practitioner and outpatient specialist care in the Netherlands: a matter of health insurance? Social Science and Medicine 1997;44(8):1161–1168.

18   Dunlop S, Coyte PC, McIsaac W. Socio-economic status and the utilisation of physicians' services: results from the Canadian National Population Health Survey. Social Science and Medicine 2000;51(1):123–133.

19   Frohlich N, Fransoo R, Roos N. Health services use in the Winnipeg Regional Health Authority: variations across areas in relation to health and socioeconomic status. Health Care Management Forum, Manitoba Centre for Health Policy 2002;Winter Supplement:9–14.

20   Veugelers PJ, Yip AM. Socioeconomic disparities in health care use: does universal coverage reduce inequalities in health? Journal of Epidemiology and Community Health 2003;57(6):424–428.

21 Castro-Leal F, Dayton J, Demery L, Mehra K. Public spending on health care in Africa: do the poor benefit? Bulletin of the World Health Organization 2000;78(1):66–74.

22 Gwatkin DR. The need for equity-oriented health sector reforms. International Journal of Epidemiology 2001;30(4):720–723.

23 Politzer RM, Yoon J, Shi L, Hughes RG, Regan J, Gaston MH. Inequality in America: the contribution of health centers in reducing and eliminating disparities in access to care. Medical Care Research and Review 2001;58(2):234–248.

24 Shi L, Regan J, Politzer RM, Luo J. Community health centers and racial/ethnic disparities in healthy life. International Journal of Health Services 2001;31(3):567–582.

25 Shi L and Starfield B. Primary care, income inequality, and self-rated health in the United States: a mixed-level analysis. International Journal of Health Services 2000;30(3):541–555.

26 Mackenbach JP. An analysis of the role of health care in reducing socioeconomic inequalities in health: the case of the Netherlands. International Journal of Health Services 2003;33(3):523–541.

27 Bryce J, el Arifeen S, Pariyo G, Lanata C, Gwatkin D, Habicht JP. Reducing child mortality: can public health deliver? Lancet 2003;362(9378):159–164.

28 Jones G, Steketee RW, Black RE, Bhutta ZA, Morris SS. How many child deaths can we prevent this year? Lancet 2003;362(9377):65–71.

29 Forrest CB, Starfield B. The effect of first-contact care with primary care clinicians on ambulatory health care expenditures. Journal of Family Practice 1996;43(1):40–48.

30 Bunker J. Medicine matters after all: measuring the benefits of medical care, a healthy lifestyle and a just social environment. London: Nuffield Trust; 2001.

31 Nolte E, McKee M. Measuring the health of nations: analysis of mortality amenable to health care. British Medical Journal 2003;327(7424):1129.

32 Starfield B. The effectiveness of primary health care. Lakhani M. A celebration of general practice. Oxon, UK: Radcliffe; 2003.

33 Goodman DC, Fisher ES, Little GA, Stukel TA, Chang CH, Schoendorf KS. The relation between the availability of neonatal intensive care and neonatal mortality. New England Journal of Medicine 2002;346(20):1538–1544.

34 Roetzheim RG, Pal N, Gonzalez EC, Ferrante JM, Van Durme DJ, Ayanian JZ, Krischer JP. The effects of physician supply on the early detection of colorectal cancer. Journal of Family Practice 1999;48(11):850–858.

35 Ferrante JM, Gonzalez EC, Pal N, Roetzheim RG. Effects of physician supply on early detection of breast cancer. Journal of the American Board of Family Practice 2000;13(6):408–414.

36 Campbell RJ, Ramirez AM, Perez K, Roetzheim RG. Cervical cancer rates and the supply of primary care physicians in Florida. Family Medicine 2003;35(1):60–64.

37 Roos NP. Who should do the surgery? Tonsillectomy-adenoidectomy in one Canadian province. Inquiry 1979;16(1):73–83.

38 Wagstaff A. Inequalities in health in developing countries: swimming against the tide? Policy Research Working Paper #2795. Washington, DC: World Bank; 2002.

39 Acheson D. Independent inquiry into inequalities in health: report. London: Stationery Office; 1998.

40 Gwatkin DR. Who would gain the most from efforts to reach the millennium development goals for health? An inquiry into the possibility of progress that fails to reach the poor. Health, Nutrition, and Population Program Discussion Paper. Washington, DC: World Bank; 2002.

41   O'Donnell O, Propper C. Equity and the distribution of UK National Health Service resources. Journal of Health Economics 1991;10(1):1–19.

42   van Doorslaer E, Wagstaff A, Rutten F. Equity in the finance and delivery of health care: an international perspective. New York: Oxford University Press; 1993.

43   Franks P, Clancy CM, Nutting PA. Gatekeeping revisited — protecting patients from overtreatment. New England Journal of Medicine 1992;327(6):424–429.

44   Wilson AJ, Oldenburg BF, Lopez AD. Targeted approaches for reducing inequities in chronic disease. Medical Journal of Australia 2003;179(5):231–232.

45   The Johns Hopkins ACG Case-Mix System Documentation Manual. Available at http://www.acg.jhsph.edu Baltimore: Health Services Research and Development Center, Johns Hopkins University; 2001.

46   Forrest CB, Majeed A, Weiner JP, Carroll K, Bindman AB. Comparison of specialty referral rates in the United Kingdom and the United States: retrospective cohort analysis. British Medical Journal 2002;325(7360):370–371.

47   Starfield B, Lemke KW, Bernhardt T, Foldes SS, Forrest CB, Weiner JP. Comorbidity: implications for the importance of primary care in 'case' management. Annals of Family Medicine 2003;1:8–14.

48   Wolff JL, Starfield B, Anderson G. Prevalence, expenditures, and complications of multiple chronic conditions in the elderly. Archives of Internal Medicine 2002;162(20):2269–2276.

49   Starfield B. Is US health really the best in the world? Journal of the American Medical Association 2000;284(4):483–485.

50   Weingart SN, Wilson RM, Gibberd RW, Harrison B. Epidemiology of medical error. British Medical Journal 2000;320(7237):774–777.

51   Himmelstein DU, Lewontin JP, Woolhandler S. Who administers? Who cares? Medical administrative and clinical employment in the United States and Canada. American Journal of Public Health 1996;86(2):172–178.

52   Woolhandler S, Himmelstein DU. Costs of care and administration at for-profit and other hospitals in the United States. New England Journal of Medicine 1997;336(11):769–774.

53   Schuster MA, McGlynn EA, Brook RH. How good is the quality of health care in the United States? Milbank Quarterly 1998;76(4):517–563, 509.

54   Kohn LT, Corrigan JM, Donaldson, MS, IOM Committee on Quality of Health Care in America. To err is human: building a safer health system. Washington DC: National Academy Press; 2000.

Section 2
Provincial/Territorial Summaries

Introduction

All Canadian provinces and territories were invited to attend the conference and to submit a summary description of their principles, progress, and future plans for transforming primary care in their jurisdictions. This section contains the summaries from the provinces and territory that submitted. Certain segments of the summaries, such as "Progress" and "Future Plans," are time specific. The reference time should be taken to be the end of 2003.

Newfoundland

PRINCIPLES

- Interdisciplinary teams (including physicians and other primary health care network providers) based on identified population needs
- Voluntary participation
- Incremental implementation, building on strengths of present system
- Integrated into regional health authorities
- Focus on wellness and community development
- Provision of services across continuum
- Enhanced access, with maximization of professional scope of practice (right service, right provider, right time)

PARTNERS

- Office of Primary Health Care to support development, implementation, and evaluation of provincial primary health care framework
- Primary Health Care Advisory Council, with provincial and stakeholder representation (i.e., associations, unions, boards) to advise the Minister re compliance of framework, its implementation and evaluation, with the provincial Strategic Health and Strategic Social Plans, and the Federal/ Provincial/Territorial direction
- Internal governmental linkages for implementation of all provincial strategies (i.e., wellness, mental health, long-term care, location of services)
- At the primary health care project level, lead VP for PHC, coordinator for PHC team, physician leader, physician network, primary health care network (public regional positions plus private health services in project area), and Local Community Advisory Committee
- Memorial University Pharmacy Liaison for clinical pharmacy support
- Newfoundland and Labrador Centre for Health Information (NLCHI) partnership for identification and implementation of electronic health record
- Partnership with provincial francophone organizations to support enhanced quality French services
- Cancer Foundation and TETRA (Telehealth and Educational Technology Resource Agency) partnership to pilot enhanced clinical use of videoconferencing

- Newfoundland and Labrador Medical Association (NLMA) PHC working group to promote formal communication with, and support enhanced relationships with, family practice physicians
- Working groups for all the identified features of primary health care framework (i.e., teams, scope of practice, emergency transportation, information management, health promotion/wellness, community capacity building, funding and payment models, governance/management) and for communication and evaluation

PROGRESS

Progress made on key elements of primary care reform:

- Provincial framework for primary health care established
- Legislation in place and updated for Nurse Practitioner, with provincial education program
- Proactively pursuing opportunities to move forward with tele-health, possibly in Atlantic partnership
- Identified person to support Office of Primary Care and NLCHI with electronic health record development and implementation

How many doctors, patients, other health care providers, regions or sites are participating?

- Regions involved: six rural and one urban, with one project in each region
- Interdisciplinary teams including physicians, nurses, other allied health professionals and some private providers (e.g., pharmacists)

SUCCESSES

- Consultation process for development of framework document involved approximately 500 stakeholders (125/425 family practice physicians)
- Presentations to stakeholders re framework document have received very positive feedback and assisted with developing momentum for primary health care renewal
- Received 24 Letters of Intent from across the province, identifying an interest to develop a proposal for primary health care based on the provincial framework (received from all but two regions of the province)
- Four of the seven projects have completed needs and service assessment for their service area, with identification of strengths and areas of improvement, have had facilitated sessions with the Office of Primary Health

Care to ensure linkages of proposal with the framework, and have submitted proposals. Funding scheduled to be provided by March 31, 2004.

- Identified evaluation process (using logic model), contracted a consultant group to support evaluation, and held initial meetings with project teams re evaluation
- Relationship-building facilitated sessions for:
  - NLMA working group
  - Institution, and Health and Community Services, Boards' CEOs, VP Medicine and Medical Officers of Health
  - PHC Advisory Council
- Several working groups have been initiated; results from working groups are being incorporated into future plans
- Started work with a communications group to develop a provincial public education campaign

CHALLENGES

- Varied health board structure across province: in two locations single board governs both institutional and community programs (integrated boards); in eight others institutional and community programs have separate boards (non-integrated boards)
- Health and Community Services have concern about loss of present good support for public health and wellness within the system with integration of teams
- Family Practice Physicians (e.g., scope of practice, autonomy, remuneration)
- Labour relation issues with providers from different organizations working in teams
- Ensuring community participation
- Connectivity issues for information management
- Operational funding for identified needed resources (e.g., human resources and teletriage)
- Evaluation (especially for health status outcomes once the transitional funding has ceased)

FUTURE PLANS

- Completion of proposal development, with project implementation, for the seven, six rural and one urban, projects
- Initiation of all working groups to support projects for sharing of successes and challenges, and assist the Office with development of provincial policy/standards/guidelines re primary health care

- Completion of evaluation plan, with implementation of monitoring and other evaluation processes, and subsequent changes to the framework as/ if appropriate
- Development of communication plan, which will include a public education strategy to inform Newfoundlanders and Labradorians about primary health care
- Work with other multi-jurisdictional and national initiatives to take advantage of successes and challenges across the country, and to maximize the resources available to the province to assist with mobilizing primary health care
- Once initial seven projects are implemented, follow up to the proposal and implementation stage with another Letter of Intent from each region of the province.

Nova Scotia

PRINCIPLES

Nova Scotia's Vision for Primary Health Care is the result of broad consultation with primary health care stakeholders, including policy and decision makers, front-line primary health care providers, and community representatives. Under the Vision the new primary health care system will be

- Community-based, family focused, and person-centred
- Comprehensive
- Responsive and flexible
- Accessible
- Integrated, collaborative, and innovative
- Accountable
- Sustainable

Some of the key strategic areas that will be pursued include

- Shifting the focus from family physicians in solo or group practice to collaborative primary health care teams involving a variety of primary health care providers
- Exploring alternatives to volume-driven funding systems for primary health care providers
- Developing a cultural shift among primary health care providers that supports a population health approach and collaboration
- Improving the integration of the primary health care system by promoting the use of Electronic Patient Record systems in primary health care organizations throughout Nova Scotia

The approach the province will take to reach this Vision will be

- Incremental and voluntary
- Through regionalized delivery by the nine District Health Authorities (DHA), consistent with the Vision and adhering to general criteria

- Rolled out differently in different communities — models will reflect community assets and needs but progressively reflect a broad primary health care approach.
- Provincial standards are being established for Primary Health Care Electronic Patient Record Systems. Standards encompass functional, technical, security, and patient privacy-related issues. Primary Health Care Organizations implementing Electronic Patient Record systems will be encouraged to select software solutions that meet provincial standards.

PARTNERS

Some structures are in place to support relationships with provider groups and other stakeholders

- As part of strengthening relationships with primary health care providers, informal meetings are in place pertaining to collaborative practice and a working group structure in place with physicians (alternate funding focus)
- The Primary Health Care Working Group is made up of district health authority representatives and is a forum for the districts (who are responsible for the delivery of primary health care services) and the Department of Health's Primary Health Care section to identify and address issues in the roll-out of system renewal.
- Building a Better Tomorrow (an Atlantic collaboration initiative) will involve the development of Education Working Groups who will be consulted and advise on the development of this change management strategy (focusing on continuing professional education of primary health care providers currently engaged in renewal activities). These Working Groups will include providers and other partners.

PROGRESS

Progress made on key elements of primary care reform:

- Registered Nurses Act and Regulations, proclaimed January 19, 2002, authorized the practice of nurse practitioners, working in collaborative practice arrangements with a physician or group of physicians anywhere in Nova Scotia
- Omnibus legislation is being developed that will provide regulatory options for groups of primary health care providers including midwives.

- NS is a partner in an Atlantic Canada collaboration focused on the development of self-care/telecare services for the region.

How many doctors, patients, other health care providers, regions or sites are participating?

- All nine District Health Authorities are participating in primary health care renewal
- Currently at proposal submission (from DHAs) and review stage
- The four Atlantic provinces are collaborating on two primary health care renewal initiatives (interdisciplinary continuing education and teletriage/ health information line).

SUCCESSES

- Successful completion of the Strengthening Primary Care in Nova Scotia Communities Initiative (under the Health Transition Fund)
- Implementation of enabling legislation for nurse practitioners
- process and development of a provincial Vision for Primary Health Care Renewal
- Process and production of the Report of the Advisory Committee on Primary Health Renewal
- Successful launch of the Diversity and Social Inclusion in Primary Health Care Initiative that will raise awareness of the needs of multicultural populations and lead to culturally inclusive guidelines and policies for the primary health care system
- Atlantic provincial collaboration

CHALLENGES

- Change management, at several levels: district/provincial governance, accountability changes; professional groups, teamwork development
- Sustainable funding
- Mechanisms for physician funding
- Public education about primary health care renewal

FUTURE PLANS

- Communication plans (to public and to health professional groups, about concepts, strategies, and goals of primary health care renewal)

- Collaborative practice and interdisciplinary team development
- Omnibus legislation, to lay foundation for primary health care models, addressing scopes of practice, collaborative practice issues
- Sustainable funding planning
- Change management initiatives
- Evaluation initiatives
- Provider education initiatives
- Guidelines for culturally competent care, addressing race, ethnicity, culture, and language
- Culturally inclusive primary health care policies, built on proposals from DHAs, and provincial strategies for nurse practitioners, midwives

Prince Edward Island

PRINCIPLES

- The Prince Edward Island Primary Health Care Redesign model is based on the principles of primary health care as defined by the World Health Organization (1978).
- One of the redesign initiatives involves the establishment of family health centres which will bring together three or more physicians, registered nurses, and other health care providers working collaboratively with shared responsibility for patient/client outcomes based on assessed health care needs. Each provider will practice to their maximum skill and competency level based on their education and experience. Physicians like all providers in the centres, will become contracted or salaried employees of the local health region, supported by improved technology. Participation by physicians is voluntary.
- A defined set of services will be provided with an emphasis on diagnosis and treatment, health promotion, illness prevention, and chronic disease management. Patients/clients will register with the family health centre, have access to extended hours of service wherever possible, and continue to see the physician of their choice, or other provider(s) depending on their presenting needs.
- Collaborative practice is fundamental to the family health centres, and will be supported through the provision of facilitation services.

PARTNERS

- A coordinator position for Primary Health Care Redesign has been established and has been positioned within the Primary Health Care Policy section of the Health Policy Development Division of the Ministry of Health & Social Services.
- A Provincial Implementation Committee has been established to oversee development of policy and strategy that support successful implementation and sustainability of PHC initiatives.
- A provincial committee of the Family Health Centre Managers has been formed to promote the implementation of a standardized model and approach to primary health care service delivery by all centres.

- Family health centre partnerships have been developed/are developing with public health nursing, speech and audiology, schools, nutrition services, addictions, mental health programs, justice, and community groups.

PROGRESS

Progress made on key elements of primary care reform.

- Nurse Practitioner legislation (in collaborative practice) is pending.
- Three of the four health centres are connected electronically to the government IHIS (health information system).
- Patient/client records have been integrated at all four health centres to enable access and sharing between appropriate providers. All physicians, nurses, alternate providers and clinical support staff at each centre are able to access and document on the patient/client files as appropriate.
- The four health centres currently offer extended hours of service from 8:00am to 8:00pm, Monday to Thursday, and 8:00am to 4:00 or 5:00pm on Friday. The hours of operation at one health centre have been extended to include weekend hours.

How many doctors, patients, other health care providers, regions or sites are participating?

- Currently, there are four family health centres being established in three health regions. (PEI has four health regions.) Each centre has a minimum approved staffing complement of 0.5 - 1.0 FTE manager, 3.0 - 4.0 FTE physicians, 2.0 FTE advanced practice nurses and administrative support. Intent is to incrementally add mental health workers and dieticians in the short-term. Over time, the skill mix of staff in each health centre will be determined by the assessed need in the community being served.

SUCCESSES

- Advance practice nurses are beginning to triage and provide follow-up for chronic disease management. Health education and information sessions/clinics are offered at specific health centres, including: audiology, asthma, blood pressure, weight checks, cholesterol reduction, footcare clinics. One health centre offers support programs (i.e., Caregiver and Tot, Breastfeeding Support), seniors programs (i.e., Walking Club,

Footcare Clinics, Yoga), and community spirit activities (i.e., Volunteer Recognition Events).
- Beechwood is the first health centre (and physician office) to install PACS, the Island-wide electronic Radiology system. The PACS system provides physicians and nurses with faster turn-around time in treating patients. X-rays are available on terminals at the centre as soon as they are completed by any radiology department at any hospital in the province. The report can be read or printed at the centre as soon as the findings are dictated.

CHALLENGES

- recruitment and retention of qualified PHC professionals
- public and health-care-provider understanding of PHC and collaborative practice
- scope of practice issues for registered nurses, doctors and nurse practitioners
- sustainability
- IT to support PHC

FUTURE PLANS

- Discussions are ongoing with other health providers who have expressed an interest in practising in a collaborative interdisciplinary environment.
- Care management protocols and/or guidelines to clarify roles, functions, and responsibilities of providers at each health centre are currently in the process of development.
- Information technology requirements specific to each health centre are being identified. Once requirements are identified, a provincial IT solution will be identified and implemented. Two priorities already identified: appointment scheduling and electronic patient/client files.

New Brunswick

PRINCIPLES

- Government of New Brunswick is committed to creating a patient-focused, community-based, integrated health services system.
- Primary health care is an important component of health care renewal in New Brunswick.
- Implementation of primary reform is mainly through regional health authorities.
- A network of Community Health Centres across the province is gradually being implemented to improve access to primary health care by providing services as close as possible to where people live.
- Objectives of CHCs are to:
  - enhance timely and appropriate access to PHC services
  - ensure citizens have 24/7 access to essential services no matter where they live
  - ensure needed affordable and reliable services are provided to defined population
  - strengthen the role of individuals, family, and community in PHC
  - enhance community health status by emphasizing health promotion, disease and injury prevention, and chronic disease management
  - establish interdisciplinary health care teams so that the most appropriate care is provided by the most appropriate provider
  - encourage linkages and collaboration among health, social, and community services

PARTNERS

- Community partnerships for determining needs/services available in Community Health Centres
- New Brunswick Medical Society-Collaborative Care Practices
- New Brunswick Nursing Association

PROGRESS

Progress made on key elements of primary care reform:

- Established the legal and regulatory framework to enable nurse practitioners to work in the NB health care system.
- Removed legislative barriers to enable an expanded role for nurses in emergency rooms.
- Removed administrative barriers to enable licensed practical nurses to work to full scope of practice.
- The introduction of a new *Health Charter of Rights and Responsibilities Bill*, to clarify for New Brunswickers what they can expect from the health system and health professionals and what the health system and health professionals can expect from them.
- The establishment of New Brunswick's first physician/nurse collaborative care practice. This collaborative practice clinic will operate seven days a week with a staff of five to six doctors, a nurse practitioner, three nurses, and two clerks. When fully staffed, the practice will provide services to the public 12 hours a day during the week and five hours each day on weekends and will serve up to 10,000 patients per year.
- Use technology to deliver services in rural/remote area, e.g., Tele-psychiatry
- The commencement (October 2002) of a new Community Health Centre network based on individual community needs identified through a community needs assessment.
- CHCs will subscribe to guiding principles:
  - provide accessible primary health care services that are culturally and linguistically appropriate
  - support individuals/communities in taking responsibility and control of their health/health care
  - collaborate, partner with other services, sectors in the community to enhance opportunities for positive health outcomes
  - focus on outcomes and evidence-based best practice delivered through interdisciplinary models of care
  - Value/support community participation in decision making
- CHCs will offer a range of comprehensive primary health care services, based on community health needs. Services are available to all residents of the Regional Health Authority with priority given to those without a family physician.
- CHCs will provide the following services:
  - assessment (individual and community level)

- health promotion and injury/disease prevention
- intervention and treatment
- referrals/consultations and partnerships
- community development related to individual and community health
- Services will be provided by a team of health care providers including physicians, nurse practitioners, nurses and other providers such as dieticians, respiratory therapists, and social workers depending on community needs

How many doctors, patients, other health care providers, regions or sites are participating?

To date four community health centres have been established in Saint John, Lameque, Doaktown, and Minto.

SUCCESSES

- Improved quality of life for health care providers working in CHCs
- More community participation and development as a result of CHCs
- Enhanced interdisciplinary teams, i.e., involving NP, OT/PT, SW, Psychology, RT, Dietician
- Collaborative Care Practice has provided enhanced and timely access to primary health care

CHALLENGES

- Health human resource shortages
- Limited funding
- Remuneration models for physicians
- Scope of practice issues
- Cultural change
- Managing public expectations of CHCs and Primary Health Care delivery models vs. traditional hospital-based models.

FUTURE PLANS

- Integrated Health Human Resources Plan
- Ambulance services enhancement
- Support of eHealth initiatives which enhance access to primary health care, e.g., telehealth

Quebec

PRINCIPLES

- Primary care network is the main foundation of the health and social services system
- Social aspect of this primary care network is the responsibility of the CLSCs (Centres locaux de services communautaires)
- Medical aspect of this primary care network is being assumed by Family Health Groups (FHGs)
- FHGs based on family physicians, in a true group practice
- Close collaboration with nurses
- Formal agreement with CLSCs
- Formal agreement with regional authorities
- Voluntary registration of patients
- Recognize and support the many doctors who already practice in the targeted manner

PARTNERS

- Ministerial Working Group (advisory)
- Ministerial Coordination Group (operational/decision making)
- Interdirectional Support Group (information and operational)

PROGRESS

Progress made on key elements of primary care reform.

- Numerous FMGs established and accredited; many more in preparation stages
- Almost full coverage of Quebec's sub-regions

How many doctors, patients, other health care providers, regions or sites are participating?

- 40 accredited FMGs; 39 more in accreditation process
- In accredited FMGs:

- 70 sites
- 417 doctors
- 39 nurses
- over 80,000 on-line registered patients, increasing at more than 3,000 each week
- 30 CLSCs

SUCCESSES

- Establishment of FMG model, and continuing growth across the province
- Implementation of patient on-line registration system
- Willingness to experiment with blended remuneration methods

CHALLENGES

- Restoration of mutual trust among doctors, CLSCs, regional authorities and Ministry
- Limitations of remuneration formulae
- Synchronization of multiple actors within the primary care network
- Modifying laws enforcing information access
- Cultural differences between urban and rural practice settings and between private and public sectors
- Need to invent new frameworks, mechanisms for cooperative interdisciplinary work

FUTURE PLANS

- Sustain political pressure
- Persevere (recognize that this is a marathon, not a sprint!)

Ontario

PRINCIPLES

- Primary health care in Ontario is patient centred.
- 24/7 access to comprehensive information, treatment, and care through a choice of a variety of models (Family Health Networks, Family Health Groups, Primary Care Networks, etc.)
- Population health approach with emphasis on prevention and promotion; and involvement of the community, i.e., focus on the broader determinants of health
- Provider participation in any of the primary health care delivery models is strictly on a voluntary basis with a choice of models.
- Access to multi/interdisciplinary teams as appropriate with clear roles and responsibilities (e.g., physicians, nurses, pharmacists, physiotherapists, social workers, and dieticians)

PARTNERS

- The Physician Services Committee (PSC) was established under the 1997 Agreement, between the Ontario government and the Ontario Medical Association, and continues under the 2000 Agreement.
- The PSC is a joint problem-solving committee that drives the implementation of the agreement between the Ontario government and physicians represented by the Ontario Medical Association through an interest-based approach including implementation issues related to primary health care.
- Through the PSC there are several working groups that allow for detailed discussion of issues and exploration of opportunities.

- The Ontario Family Health Network (OFHN) was established in March 2001 to facilitate and manage the implementation of Family Health Networks in Ontario and provide advice to the Minister of Health and Long-Term Care.
- The implementation activities of the Ontario Family Health Network agency are carried out and managed by the chair and chief executive officer who in turn report to the OFHN Board. The OFHN Board has 14 members comprised of the chair, representatives from the Ontario Medical

Association, health care providers, the business community, the regulatory colleges, health experts, and the public.

- OFHN staff assists physicians who have expressed an interest in establishing a Family Health Network or Family Health Group in their community by providing details of the model, calculating their estimated projected revenue, and through a number of support mechanisms to assist with group formation and patient enrolment.

- Several advisory committees have been established that include all colleges and associations for the primary health care regulated health professions to provide advice on the use of federal one-time funding and with the Academic Health Science Centres to discuss opportunities for research and evaluation.

PROGRESS

Progress made on key elements of primary care reform:

- Ontario has legislation in place for all primary health care providers through the Regulated Health Professions Act. Specific legislation has been passed for RN(EC)s (nurse practitioners).
- Ontario has established an ePhysician Health Council to develop acceptable tools, architecture, security and support for the implementation of electronic medical records and decision support tools. $150 M in one-time funding has been allocated to support this.
- Currently, an integrated telephone health advisory service is being implemented that links after hours, weekend, and holiday advice with an on-call physician in each of the primary care models and provides for next-day report back on the nature of calls.
- A large systems project is in place to facilitate the development and implementation of funding and enrolment processes.

How many doctors, patients, other health care providers, regions or sites are participating?

- As of January 2004, there are 2,415 physicians participating in 318 primary care delivery group models. These include: Family Health Networks, Family Health Groups, Health Service Organizations, Primary Care Networks, Northern Group Funding Plans, Community Sponsored Contracts, Community Health Centres, and the Group Health Centre.

SUCCESSES

- Primary Care Networks (which were the original pilot models), Family Health Networks, Family Health Groups, Health Service Organizations, Community Health Centres, and the Group Health Centre are all considered to be successful primary health care delivery models.
- Alignment of the "existing" primary care delivery models (Health Service Organizations, Primary Care Networks) to the "newer" models (i.e., Family Health Networks, Family Health Groups) to harmonize core elements such as: patient enrolment, after hours requirements, comprehensive care descriptions, access to Telephone Health Advisory Service and information technology, introduction of population-based incentives and comprehensive care incentives, and equity in compensation (across capitation models).
- Fall 2002 announcement of 369 nurse practitioner positions in underserviced and rural communities. In May 2003, 117 positions were awarded in small, rural and underserviced communities.
- A positive working relationship and "partnership" with the medical association.

CHALLENGES

- Integration of other interdisciplinary providers into primary health care settings (challenges include ongoing funding, collaborative practice models, and liability issues)
- Growing concern about the availability of a sufficient number of primary health care providers
- Community involvement/engagement and ownership models
- Administrative burden — for physicians, other providers and the ministry
- Lack of infrastructure funding and support
- Time it takes to effect change — including implementation of information technology

FUTURE PLANS

- The Government of Ontario plans to deliver better family health care through 150 family health teams. Family Health Teams will not be a top down, one-size-fits-all approach. The government will partner with communities in building Family Health Teams to meet their needs.
- The Ontario Government will be entering into negotiations with the Ontario Medical Association to negotiate a new Framework Agreement for physicians in January 2004.

Manitoba

PRINCIPLES

In Manitoba, the approach to primary health care reform involved promoting, innovative, needs-based primary health care initiatives and implementing small incremental but positive changes to primary health care service delivery. Since 2001 significant activity has occurred in the following areas:

- A current state assessment of primary health care within the province was completed to assist in the development of policy.
- An interdepartmental team was struck to develop a Primary Health Care Policy Framework (PHCPF) which would outline the direction upon which to develop and evolve primary health care within the Province of Manitoba.
- The PHCPF assisted in the strategic use of the Primary Health Care Transition Fund, Provincial Envelope enabling Manitoba to outline a two-phased approach. Phase one involved supporting provincial initiatives that address barriers to the development and implementation of primary health care. These initiatives included: development of a provincial health call centre; development of a collaborative practice training program; development of information technology to integrate health information and provide appropriate timely access to the benefit of the client and health care provider; development of a public awareness campaign; skill enhancements of emergency service providers in rural and northern Manitoba.
- Phase two of the PHCPF Provincial Envelope supported initiatives identified by the Regional Health Authorities (RHAs) that facilitate and foster development of primary health care specific to the needs of the RHA. This was accomplished by soliciting a call for proposals based upon selection criteria and guidelines which embodied Health Canada's and Manitoba Health's policy guidelines on primary health care reform. Seventeen proposals were selected. Each RHA had a minimum of one PHC initiative approved for funding.

PROGRESS

Progress made on key elements of primary care reform:

- Manitoba Health has been successful in supporting legislation for Midwifery and Advance Practice Nursing.
- Seventeen RHA-led primary health care initiatives have been supported by Manitoba Health through the PHCPF – Phase Two initiatives. These initiatives were selected based on their ability to support advancing primary care access (family physicians and advance practice nursing), building community capacity, increasing regional health authority organizational strength, and creating integrated service delivery systems.
- Construction of the provincial health call centre (Health Links) has been completed. A soft launch to provide real time service response to callers is now being implemented.

How many doctors, patients, other health care providers, regions or sites are participating?

- Each Regional Health Authority received funding for at least one of their PHC initiatives to move PHC forward specific to the region's needs and capabilities. All initiatives are underway to varying degrees.

SUCCESSES

- The establishment of a provincial telephone triage/health call centre has enabled Manitoba citizens, through the use of telephone technology, to gain timely access to heath information and advice on health concerns. This provides Manitoba citizens with information and options on how to best access the health system to meet their needs.

CHALLENGES

- Development of financial remuneration models that enable PHC service providers to deliver services in ways that reflect PHC principles.
- Development and establishment of PHC providers who are appropriately trained for practice in an integrated, interdisciplinary service delivery setting.
- The introduction and implementation of effective information technology that supports interdisciplinary PHC teams through the continuum of care.

- Change management to facilitate evolution of existing regional health delivery systems to primary health care service delivery models.

FUTURE PLANS

- To review, analyze, and recommend changes to the existing PHC policy framework to ensure the policy continues to drive activity and development of PHC within the province. This exercise involves consultation with internal and external stakeholders in PHC to remain relevant and achievable within the regions.
- Planning and discussion to lead to development of financial remuneration models.

Saskatchewan

PRINCIPLES

The Saskatchewan approach to primary health care reform began with *Caring for Medicare*. From this review, *The Action Plan for Saskatchewan Health* and *The Action Plan for Primary Health Care* were developed. The key initiatives in the action plan were:

- The development of an integrated system of health services on a 24/7/ 365 basis delivered through regional health authorities (RHAs) in managed networks with teams of health care providers.
- Goal of teams established to provide accessibility to 25 percent of the population in four years and 100 percent of the population in ten years.
- The overarching principles are those of quality and access.

The Action Plan for Primary Health Care was based on the following characteristics:

- securing a defined population (each RHA will provide a core set of primary health care services to a defined population);
- client services (clients will be able to choose their health care provider);
- integration of services (a range of coordinated services including health promotion, prevention, primary curative care, rehabilitative and supportive care — provided by multidisciplinary teams);
- community participation and development (role for communities in the development of primary health care);
- defined access and service standards;
- a human resources continuum; and
- non-fee-for-service remuneration for GPs.

Saskatchewan has 21 demonstration sites that have been developed and is in the process of evaluating them. The evaluation will form the basis of ongoing primary health developments.

PARTNERS

- Regular meetings between Primary Health Services Branch (Department of Health) and stakeholder groups (Saskatchewan Medical Association [SMA], regulatory bodies, and union groups).
- Regular meetings with the Integrated Primary Health Care Working Group (multi-stakeholder group).
- Meetings with the Primary Care Working Group of the SMA.
- Hiring directors of Primary Health Care to work within the RHAs to co-ordinate development of primary health care.
- Regular meeting with the directors of Primary Health Care.
- Development of primary health care plans by each RHA.
- Establishment of broad-based steering committees in each RHA to de-velop and implement primary health care plans.

PROGRESS

Progress made on key elements of primary care reform:

- RHA Primary Health Care Plans have been developed.
- Registered Nurse (Nurse Practitioner) legislation has been passed; by-laws have been signed; regulations are close to sign off recognizing the role of the RN(NP); anticipated date for RN(NP) licensure – April 1, 2004.
- Ongoing discussions with the Saskatchewan Medical Association regard-ing alternate funding models and team formation.
- HealthLine established August 2003.
- Provincial Information Technology (IT) Strategy developed with primary health care IT a major component.

How many doctors, patients, other health care providers, regions or sites are participating?

- At present there are 24 primary health care teams in Saskatchewan with the core of the teams being general practitioners (GPs) and nurse practi-tioners (NPs). The 24 teams involve 80 GPs and 24 NPs serving 80,000 – 100,000 clients.

SUCCESSES

- HealthLine
- RHA Primary Health Care Plans developed
- Directors of Primary Health Care present in RHAs
- Team Development strategy successful in pilot phase
- Nurse Practitioner Licensure
- Liaison with stakeholder groups ongoing

CHALLENGES

- Sustained funding for primary health care
- Change management challenges for health providers
- Appropriate IT development
- Liability issues for health providers
- Scope of practice challenges for health providers

FUTURE PLANS

- Agreement on GP funding models
- Health accord dollars allocated for team development within RHAs
- RHA level evaluation document
- Province-wide facilitation strategy for team development
- Standard development for primary health care IT

Alberta

PRINCIPLES

- Focus on primary care as starting point
- Facilitating and creating the incentive for partnerships between the regional health authorities and physicians to provide a range of defined primary care services
- Voluntary participation by physicians
- Best practice based on pilot initiatives funded over the past five years

PARTNERS

- A key relationship has been established with the Alberta Medical Association and the Regional Health Authorities through the recent tripartite AMA agreement which includes a primary care agreement outlining the process, requirements, and incentives for regional health authorities and physicians to form local primary care initiatives (LPCIs).
- This agreement is governed by a tripartite committee structure consisting of a master committee, a secretariat and four sub-committees for each of the key sub-agreements: Physician Office System Program (POSP), Physician Services, Physician On Call Program, and the Primary Care Initiative.

PROGRESS

Progress made on key elements of primary care reform:

- The *Health Professions Act* replaces exclusive scope of practice with a system of overarching scope of practice regulations that operate in conjunction with a schedule of restricted activities set out in the *Government Organization Act*. Regulations will specify which activities may be carried out by members of regulated health professions and set out continued competency programs for each profession.
- The Alberta Electronic Health Record (EHR) is a province-wide clinical health information system that links physicians, pharmacists, hospitals, home care, and other providers across the province. The record stores pertinent patient information on-line so that health care providers may

access a patient's prescription history, allergies, and laboratory test results immediately on-line.
- The implementation of the province-wide health advice and information service, Health Link Alberta, provides all Albertans with 24/7 access to credible health information, advice, referral, and information about finding services.
- Provision of Alternate Payment Plan (ARP) options for physicians.
- Per capita funding to local primary care initiatives for individuals formally or informally rostered will enable the partners in these service agreements to provide enhanced primary care services.
- Capital funding through the Health Sustainability Initiative to support capital infrastructure costs related to primary health care reform.

How many doctors, patients, other health care providers, regions or sites are participating?

- This initiative is new – the target is to approve 12 letters of intent across the province by June 2004; ultimately all Albertans should have the opportunity to belong to a LPCI.

SUCCESSES

- Tripartite AMA primary care agreement
- Electronic Health Record
- Health Professions Act legislation
- Health Link Alberta

CHALLENGES

- Public awareness and support
- Developing a culture of partnership and collaboration
- Ensuring that other health providers and health professionals understand the opportunities and participate in the initiative

FUTURE PLANS

- Provincial roll-out of LPCIs over the next two-plus years

British Columbia

PRINCIPLES

- Ministry of Health/Health Authority partnership: ministry sets policy; health authorities plan and implement.
- Flexible range of practice models available, based on provincially prescribed principles, including Primary Health Care Organizations (PHCO), Community Health Centres (CHC), Patient Care Network (PCN), Shared Care, and different levels of engagement, i.e., "one size does not fit all."
- Voluntary: physician practices self-select to participate in initiatives. Health authorities employ different methods to recruit physicians to participate in new models.
- Multi-disciplinary practice is encouraged. PHCOs, CHCs, and Shared Care arrangements rely on physicians, specialists, nurses, and allied health professionals working in teams.
- Accountable: health authorities (7) are responsible for the implementation of the initiatives identified in their Ministry of Health approved Primary Health Care Transition Fund (PHCTF) plans.
- Sustainable: all initiatives implemented under the health authorities' PHCTF plans must be self-sustaining by March 2006.

PARTNERS

- Health authorities: provide oversight and implementation of projects identified in their PHCTF plans. These functions are achieved via coordinating committees with administrative/clinical representation.
- Provincial Steering Committee: provides advice and guidance on current and future primary health care renewal programs and policies. The committee consists of provincial Ministry of Health, health authorities, professional organizations, and academic representatives.
- Working Committees: provide technical and operational advice on project implementation, program development, and evaluation. Membership consists of health authority administrative and clinical representatives.
- Chronic Disease Management (CDM) collaboratives: consist of physician-led primary health care teams engaged in the development and delivery

of care based on established clinical guidelines for diseases such as diabetes, congestive heart failure, and depression.
- Ministry of Health: Primary Health Care Branch provides provincial level coordination and support to the health authorities. In its capacity as steward, the branch provides implementation support, evaluation, and monitoring of plan implementation.

PROGRESS

Progress made on key elements of primary care reform:

- A blended funding formula for PHCOs has been established and refined. This funding model consists of a blend of capitated funding for core services and fee-for-service funding for non-core services. The capitated funding is based upon a patient's adjusted clinical group, age, and sex (John Hopkin's ACG model). Non-core services include obstetrics and anaethesia. PHCOs have the opportunity to increase their revenue by increasing the number of patients using their practice.
- Enabling legislation for nurse practitioners (NP) was passed this fall. Work is currently underway to define the scope of practice for NPs, which will be described in the regulations under the *Health Practitioners' Act.*
- Electronic Medical Summary, which will provide an overview of critical clinical and laboratory information in a form that can follow a patient through the medical system, is under development.
- Integration of information technology in clinical practices, using recommended provincial performance standards.

How many doctors, patients, other health care providers, regions or sites are participating?

All seven health authorities are participating. Review of health authority PHCTF plans indicates that there has been engagement in the full spectrum of practice models (PHCOs, CHCs, PCNs, and Shared Care).

- Based upon the PHCTF plan reviews up to 30 primary health care sites or initiatives are expected to be established province-wide.
- Three CDM collaboratives have been established. Two province-wide collaboratives for congestive heart failure (CHF) and diabetes. The CHF collaborative involves 40 physician-led teams; whereas the diabetes collaborative involves 70 physician-led teams. A regional diabetes, CHF, and

depression collaborative involving 30 physician-led teams has been established on Vancouver Island.

- It is anticipated that three more collaboratives will be established over the next two years that will involve as many as 650 additional physician-led teams.
- The General Practice Service Committee has also established a CDM initiative in which over 1,000 physicians throughout the province are participating.
- The CDM Toolkit has been created as an extension of the ministry's Secure Web Site for Practitioners. It offers a range of functions including web-based access to clinical guidelines for treating conditions such as diabetes, depression and congestive heart failure. It lets practitioners complete patient flowsheets electronically — automatically integrating relevant clinical guidelines. There are currently 450 physicians registered with the CDM Toolkit and the number of users is anticipated to increase to between 1,000 and 1,500 practitioners by March 2005.

SUCCESSES

- Partnership with the health authorities to take on lead responsibility for primary health care renewal during a period of health authority redesign.
- Health authorities have planned for a broad range of options/models for primary health care renewal.
- Work with University of British Columbia to develop administrative data for the evaluation of primary health care initiatives.
- Development of patient care guidelines, secure patient registry and quality improvement collaboratives for chronic disease management.
- Addition of pharmacist services to the *BC* Nurseline, which is a 24/7 telephone triage service provided by RNs.
- Educational workshops to support change management, clinical practice redesign, and multi-disciplinary practice. Semi-annual primary health care sites workshops to exchange information on emerging issues or concerns.
- Communication/public information materials: PHCTF Newsletter, PHCO Bulletins, Primary Health Care Website.

CHALLENGES

- Physician and provider remuneration/limited funding and compensation models
- Health care system focus on acute care

- Fragmentation of health care delivery/system
- Scope of practice issues
- Resistance to change, at system level and provider practice level
- Integration of information technology (technical aspects, funding, and provider acceptance)

FUTURE PLANS

- Continued support for the health authorities as they implement primary health care planned initiatives.
- Development of a provincial primary health care policy framework.
- Continued work on a provincial evaluation framework.
- Second provincial primary health care educational conference and various workshops to support change management, clinical practice redesign, and multi-disciplinary teams.

Yukon Territory

PRINCIPLES

The general approach being taken by the Government of Yukon is

- Building on existing programs and organizations, to strengthen the coordination and integration of government and non-government activities that improve population health.

PARTNERS

To date, relationships and structures include those listed below:

- Primary Health Care Transition Fund unit comprising a coordinator and policy analyst
- Steering committee within Department of Health and Social Services to provide direction to unit
- Involvement of stakeholders in planning process, including environmental scan and PHC planning forum. Stakeholders included representatives of professions, federal, territorial, municipal and First Nations governments, non-government organizations, and the general public.

Further planning may lead to the creation of temporary structures and ongoing relationships for implementation of reforms.

PROGRESS

Progress made on key elements of primary care reform:

- Initial actions are underway, including initiatives for providing health information to the public, supporting healthy living (prevention of chronic disease), addressing the priority health issue of substance abuse, and doing preliminary work to improve case-information sharing among primary health care programs. Improved information on use of ambulatory care services is being collected. Planning for implementation of information technology improvements has commenced.

How many doctors, patients, other health care providers, regions or sites are participating?

- Varies with actions. This question cannot be answered in the same way for the Yukon as it can for provinces/territories that are moving to some new form of primary health care organization. We are working to improve coordination within and among existing programs without putting different organizational structures in place.

SUCCESSES

- Primary Health Care Planning forum involving multiple stakeholders

CHALLENGES

- Policy and process for case information sharing
- Building capacity within the system and at the individual level for improved health outcomes
- Sustainability of change beyond end of PHCTF funding period

FUTURE PLANS

- Further development of plans based on information from environmental scan, planning forum, and literature review.

Contributors

Marie-Dominique Beaulieu, Professor, Dr. Sadok Besrour Chair in Family Medicine, Research Centre of the Centre hospitalier de l'université de Montréal and University of Montreal

Jackie Cumming, Director, Health Services Research, Victoria University of Wellington

Raisa Deber, Professor, Health Policy, Management and Evaluation, University of Toronto

Michael Decter, Chairman, Health Council of Canada

John Dorland, Assistant Professor, Community Health and Epidemiology, Queen's University; Evaluation Program, Ontario Family Health Network

Cathy Fooks, Director, Health Network, Canadian Policy Research Networks

Brian Hutchison, Director, Centre for Health Economics and Policy Analysis, McMaster University; Professor, Departments of Family Medicine and Clinical Epidemiology and Biostatistics, McMaster University

Antonia Maioni, Director, McGill Institute for the Study of Canada, Associate Professor of Political Science and William Dawson Scholar, McGill University

Nicholas Mays, Professor of Health Policy, Department of Public Health and Policy, London School of Hygiene and Tropical Medicine, University of London; part-time Principal Adviser, Health and Cross-Sector Strategy Sections, Social Policy Branch, New Zealand Treasury

Martin Roland, Professor of General Practice; Director of the National Primary Care Research and Development Centre, University of Manchester

Rod Sheaff, Senior Research Fellow, National Primary Care Research and Development Centre, University of Manchester

S.E.D. Shortt, Director, Centre for Health Services and Policy Research, Queen's University

Bonnie Sibbald, Professor, Health Services Research; Deputy Director, National Primary Care Research and Development Centre, University of Manchester

Barbara Starfield, Professor, Health Policy and Management, Johns Hopkins University

Carolyn Hughes Tuohy, Vice President, Policy Development, Associate Provost, University of Toronto

Ruth Wilson, Professor, Family Medicine, Queen's University; Chair, Ontario Family Health Network

Queen's Policy Studies
Recent Publications

The Queen's Policy Studies Series is dedicated to the exploration of major policy issues that confront governments in Canada and other western nations. McGill-Queen's University Press is the exclusive world representative and distributor of books in the series.

School of Policy Studies

Social and Cultural Change, David Last, Franklin Pinch, Douglas L. Bland and Alan Okros (eds.), 2004 Paper ISBN 1-55339-032-6 Cloth 1-55339-033-4

Clusters in a Cold Climate: Innovation Dynamics in a Diverse Economy, David A. Wolfe and Matthew Lucas (eds.), 2004 Paper ISBN 1-55339-038-5 Cloth 1-55339-039-3

Canada Without Armed Forces? Douglas L. Bland (ed.), 2004
Paper ISBN 1-55339-036-9 Cloth 1-55339-037-7

Campaigns for International Security: Canada's Defence Policy at the Turn of the Century, Douglas L. Bland and Sean M. Maloney, 2004
Paper ISBN 0-88911-962-7 Cloth 0-88911-964-3

Understanding Innovation in Canadian Industry, Fred Gault (ed.), 2003
Paper ISBN 1-55339-030-X Cloth ISBN 1-55339-031-8

Delicate Dances: Public Policy and the Nonprofit Sector, Kathy L. Brock (ed.), 2003
Paper ISBN 0-88911-953-8 Cloth ISBN 0-88911-955-4

Beyond the National Divide: Regional Dimensions of Industrial Relations, Mark Thompson, Joseph B. Rose and Anthony E. Smith (eds.), 2003
Paper ISBN 0-88911-963-5 Cloth ISBN 0-88911-965-1

The Nonprofit Sector in Interesting Times: Case Studies in a Changing Sector, Kathy L. Brock and Keith G. Banting (eds.), 2003
Paper ISBN 0-88911-941-4 Cloth ISBN 0-88911-943-0

Clusters Old and New: The Transition to a Knowledge Economy in Canada's Regions, David A. Wolfe (ed.), 2003 Paper ISBN 0-88911-959-7 Cloth ISBN 0-88911-961-9

The e-Connected World: Risks and Opportunities, Stephen Coleman (ed.), 2003
Paper ISBN 0-88911-945-7 Cloth ISBN 0-88911-947-3

Knowledge, Clusters and Regional Innovation: Economic Development in Canada, J. Adam Holbrook and David A. Wolfe (eds.), 2002
Paper ISBN 0-88911-919-8 Cloth ISBN 0-88911-917-1

Lessons of Everyday Law/Le droit du quotidien, Roderick Alexander Macdonald, 2002
Paper ISBN 0-88911-915-5 Cloth ISBN 0-88911-913-9

Improving Connections Between Governments and Nonprofit and Voluntary Organizations: Public Policy and the Third Sector, Kathy L. Brock (ed.), 2002
Paper ISBN 0-88911-899-X Cloth ISBN 0-88911-907-4

Institute of Intergovernmental Relations

Canada: The State of the Federation 2002, vol. 16, *Reconsidering the Institutions of Canadian Federalism*, J. Peter Meekison, Hamish Telford and Harvey Lazar (eds.), 2004
Paper ISBN 1-55339-009-1 Cloth ISBN 1-55339-008-3

Federalism and Labour Market Policy: Comparing Different Governance and Employment Strategies, Alain Noël (ed.), 2004
Paper ISBN 1-55339-006-7 Cloth ISBN 1-55339-007-5

The Impact of Global and Regional Integration on Federal Systems: A Comparative Analysis, Harvey Lazar, Hamish Telford and Ronald L. Watts (eds.), 2003
Paper ISBN 1-55339-002-4 Cloth ISBN 1-55339-003-2

Canada: The State of the Federation 2001, vol. 15, *Canadian Political Culture(s) in Transition*, Hamish Telford and Harvey Lazar (eds.), 2002
Paper ISBN 0-88911-863-9 Cloth ISBN 0-88911-851-5

Federalism, Democracy and Disability Policy in Canada, Alan Puttee (ed.), 2002
Paper ISBN 0-88911-855-8 Cloth ISBN 1-55339-001-6, ISBN 0-88911-845-0 (set)

Comparaison des régimes fédéraux, 2ᵉ éd., Ronald L. Watts, 2002
ISBN 1-55339-005-9

John Deutsch Institute for the Study of Economic Policy

The 2003 Federal Budget: Conflicting Tensions, Charles M. Beach and Thomas A. Wilson (eds.), 2004   Paper ISBN 0-88911-958-9 Cloth ISBN 0-88911-956-2

Canadian Immigration Policy for the 21st Century, Charles M. Beach, Alan G. Green and Jeffrey G. Reitz (eds.), 2003   Paper ISBN 0-88911-954-6 Cloth ISBN 0-88911-952-X

Framing Financial Structure in an Information Environment, Thomas J. Courchene and Edwin H. Neave (eds.), Policy Forum Series no. 38, 2003
Paper ISBN 0-88911-950-3 Cloth ISBN 0-88911-948-1

Towards Evidence-Based Policy for Canadian Education/Vers des politiques canadiennes d'éducation fondées sur la recherche, Patrice de Broucker and/et Arthur Sweetman (eds./dirs.), 2002 Paper ISBN 0-88911-946-5 Cloth ISBN 0-88911-944-9

Money, Markets and Mobility: Celebrating the Ideas of Robert A. Mundell, Nobel Laureate in Economic Sciences, Thomas J. Courchene (ed.), 2002
Paper ISBN 0-88911-820-5 Cloth ISBN 0-88911-818-3

Available from: McGill-Queen's University Press
c/o Georgetown Terminal Warehouses
34 Armstrong Avenue
Georgetown, Ontario L7G 4R9
Tel: (877) 864-8477
Fax: (877) 864-4272
E-mail: orders@gtwcanada.com